Man-Living-Health:
A Theory of Nursing

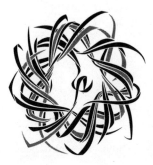

ROSEMARIE RIZZO PARSE, PH.D., R.N.
Pittsburgh, Pennsylvania

81787

A WILEY MEDICAL PUBLICATION
JOHN WILEY & SONS
New York • Chichester • Brisbane • Toronto

Cover and interior design by Wanda Lubelska.
Logo by Alj Mary.

Library of Congress Cataloging in Publication Data:

Parse, Rosemarie Rizzo.
  Man-living-health.

  Bibliography: p.
  Includes index.
  1. Nursing—Philosophy. I. Title. [DNLM:
1. Philosophy, Nursing. WY 86 P266m]

RT84.5.P36   610.73'01   81-219
ISBN 0-471-04443-1   AACR2

Printed in the United States of America

10 9 8 7 6 5 4 3 2 1

THE LORD GOD FORMED MAN OUT OF THE CLAY OF THE GROUND AND BLEW INTO HIS NOSTRILS THE BREATH OF LIFE, AND SO MAN BECAME A LIVING BEING.

Gen. 2:7-9.

Prologue

THE *TRUTH* OF CERTAIN EMPIRICAL PROPOSITIONS BE-
LONGS TO OUR FRAME OF REFERENCE.

Ludwig Wittgenstein

Nursing is moving toward its place in the academic sun as a scholarly discipline whose science is just beginning to blossom. Science is a quest for truth and knowledge. It does not purport to find *the* truth but rather many truths. The emphasis, therefore, is on the quest. Sir Karl Popper emphasizes this distinction in his discussion of "the path of science." He says that "the wrong view of science betrays itself in the craving to be right; for it is not his possession of knowledge of irrefutable truth that makes the man of science, but his persistent and recklessly critical *quest* for truth."[1] According to Popper, then, the path of science is the route of inquiry, of questioning and of questing for knowledge. The truth and knowledge as it unfolds from scientific questing is always rooted in a set of assumptions. The quotation from Ludwig Wittgenstein that opens this prologue further emphasizes the point of view that scientific truths are constituted in one's frame of reference.

As nursing evolves its theories, it is important that they be critically examined for their contribution to the developing science of nursing. In this infancy of scientific development, theories will be proposed in

[1] Sir Karl Popper, *The Logic of Scientific Discovery*, 3rd edition (London: Hutchinson Publishing Company, 1968), pp. 280-281.

parallel fashion or may evolve genealogically, that is, be generated from existing conceptual frameworks in nursing. How ever they are created, it is a necessary criterion of evaluation that each be questioned in light of the frame of reference from which it is proposed.

Man-Living-Health: A Theory of Nursing is based on explicitly stated assumptions and logically developed within the themes that emerge from these assumptions. The theory proposes a way of looking at man and health that enlarges the emerging science of nursing. The frame of reference of this theory is grounded in the image of science as a process. Science has been defined as a process and a product. Generally, however, it is conceived as a body of laws derived from observable data that have been organized and classified for the purpose of explaining and predicting events in nature. This understanding of science suggests a certain priority in technological application or science as product. While the idea of science as process is not new, it is less valued in a technological society that is product-oriented.

However, historians and philosophers of science continue to debate and defend science as process. As early as 1938, Leslie White proposed that, although the word *science* is a noun implying a thing or state, it is appropriate to use it as a verb with its connotation of activity. In his article, "Science is Sciencing," he says, "Science is not merely a collection of facts and formulas. It is preeminently a way of dealing with experience. The word may be appropriately used as a verb: one sciences; i.e., deals with experience according to certain assumptions and with certain techniques."[2] With these words, Leslie White calls out the fundamental essence of science as a human activity. Basic to his point of view is the premise that science offers one the opportunity to know the world through a process of discovery. Consistent with

[2] Leslie A. White, "Science Is Sciencing," *Philosophy of Science*, 5(4), October 1938, pp. 369–389.

Wittgenstein, White suggests that this process of discovery is rooted in a particular way of thinking about the world, because he explicitly states that one "sciences" based on certain assumptions. In this sense, sciencing is a dynamic activity concerned with the generic process of coming to know in contradistinction to science as product culminating in technology. According to White, it is the very essence of sciencing to interrelate particular phenomena of man's experience within a system of beliefs and to design the techniques appropriate to that system. Science conceptualized as a noun or product values *answers*, whereas sciencing conceptualized as a verb or process places value on the questions raised and the methods designed to generate new insights and new concepts. This does not imply that sciencing does not also seek answers; it does. The answers, however, are pathways to new questions that are heuristic and generate new avenues for questing. The verb and noun forms of the word *science* are not meant to create a dichotomy but rather to illuminate the intricate complexity of the interaction of science as parent of technology and sciencing as generic process of coming to know. The way of science, then, is multifaceted, yet its many profiles reveal a common theme. This theme is recognized in the language of science, which includes ways of describing as well as explaining and predicting phenomena. In the process of sciencing, describing phenomena enhances one's way of giving meaning to the world. This language addresses the very core of sciencing as a problem-solving activity, whether in the sense of questing for abstract knowing, searching for applied outcomes, or both. This multifaceted way of science, then, shows itself as a complex interrelationship that structures the science and the sciencing.

The complementary nature of the science-sciencing interrelationship sometimes becomes obscured as an academic discipline moves toward maturity as a science. The structure of science connects the rational and the intuitive, the empirical and the theoretical, the thought and the practice in the generic process of sciencing. It is within this structure of science as sciencing that this theory Man-Living-Health enlarges the emerging science of nursing.

As the discipline of nursing develops its science, a continuing quest is that of defining its unique body of knowledge: a body of knowledge knowable only in the formal study of nursing. One of the criteria for uniqueness in the body of knowledge is that of differentiation. The discipline of nursing defines its uniqueness through differentiating itself in light of other health disciplines. It is important to remember that the boundaries that separate disciplines are tenuous and yielding. Nursing shares a focus with medicine, psychology, and social work, among others, in that all these disciplines study man and health. The relationship of nursing to these disciplines, then, can be examined in light of the organizational structure and the substance of the conceptual framework that guides the proper object of inquiry. Some overlap among disciplines is to be expected in light of the universe of discourse of all human knowledge as well as the partial universe of discourse chosen by each health discipline as its own object of inquiry. The organizational structure of each discipline defines the relationship and the patterning of the concepts relative to man and health. As the structure of the question is examined, the distinctness in each discipline unfolds as the substance of the conceptual framework comes into focus. The substantive difference is mainly in the philosophic framework of the worldview espoused, which is most evident in the basic assumptions about man and health and the predominant themes that emerge from them. It is these assumptions, whether implicit or explicit, that guide the characterization of the phenomena to be studied by each discipline. It follows that the methods chosen for study and the findings that are uncovered will be in light of these basic assumptions. One can examine the major focus of the scholarly pursuits of health disciplines and can conclude that, while the content chosen for study may be similar, the structure, the process, and the results are quite different. For example, medicine is concerned with man and health predominantly through emphasis on the prevention and cure of disease. In light of this focus, the starting point of inquiry for the discipline of medicine is disease. Psychology, in its study of man, has as its frame of reference psychological processes that address mental abilities and adjustments. The starting point of inquiry for psychology is man's emotional responses. Nursing, in its study of man, has as its frame of reference patterns of living health. The starting point of inquiry for nursing relative to man and health is the interhuman processes of caring and healing.

The values and characteristics of the disciplines just named illuminate the coherence of the conceptual system that particularizes and differentiates the disciplines from each other. Viewed in this way, the overlap of questions chosen for study is seen to yield a richer, more diverse, and complementary understanding of man and health. Admittedly, then, there is conceptual overlap, and the boundaries that separate the disciplines one from the other are tenuous at best, yet identifable, for it is the worldview that guides the intellectual questions pursued by each discipline that creates the differentiation among them. It is the way in which the phenomenal world is synthesized with the nuomenal world that will propel the emergence of nursing as a scholarly, scientific endeavor into the twenty-first century.

This book has created such a synthesis. It builds on the rich traditions of nursing's historical involvement with man, health, and environment. The theory develops these traditional concepts consistent with an ideological perspective that illuminates them in a unique way.

Some of the predominant ideas that emerge from this

work and give rise to the questions that will be the starting point of inquiry are:

- Man as experiencing subject
- Interconnected evolution of man and world
- Health as becoming process
- Nature of change as ongoing and participative

These ideas surface throughout the theoretical presentation as the assumptions are developed in the text. Consistent with White's notion of sciencing, these assumptions and the theory Man-Living-Health that unfolds from them demonstrate value for the questions that will be raised in light of new insights and new concepts. These new insights will further develop the theory of Man-Living-Health as individual nurses who come to know the theory engage in the research required to generate the new concepts. The science of an academic discipline builds through time in patterned stages toward maturity through the rigors of research. This research is grounded in a conceptual system that unfolds from a particular view of the world. Rosemarie Rizzo Parse, in creating this theory, has expressed truth for her through the sharing of a particular worldview about man and health for the discipline of nursing. In so doing, she has lived the ideal of what might be for nursing. The influence of this thinking has already made a difference to those who have been touched by it. I invite the reader to see and to hear the printed words and to dwell with the thoughts and feelings that unfold in being with them. It is in this dwelling that new possibilities for nursing surface on each reader's unique horizon.

TRUTH EXISTS FOR THE INDIVIDUAL ONLY AS HE HIMSELF PRODUCES IT IN ACTION.

Kierkegaard

A. Barbara Coyne, Ph.D., R.N.

Preface

There is an alive and growing force within nursing today generating energy toward the advancement of nursing as a scientific discipline. This book articulates a theory of nursing which supports this growing force.

The intent of this work is to set forth a different paradigm of nursing, a theory rooted in the human sciences, an alternative to the traditional. The different paradigm is the theory of nursing as Man*-Living-Health. This theory was genealogically created to enhance nursing's unique body of knowledge. The idea to create such a theory began many years ago when I began to wonder and wander and ask why not?

The theory itself, as articulated in this book, surfaced in me in Janusian fashion over the years in interrelationship with others primarily through my lived experience with nursing. The creation of it has been long and arduous, but with many moments of joy. The components have been seen, at times, as through a glass darkly. They have been elusive, abstract, and disparate—and often, just beyond my reach. To present the theory in this book appears to say "it is finished!" Yet the theory has only just begun to be viewed and enhanced by those who take up the challenge to evolve nursing science to a higher level of complexity and specificity. While the written theory follows in the pages of this book, the

*Man, throughout the text, refers to *homo sapiens.*

nuances and mysteries of it continue to stir in me new ideas, yet different ways of viewing Man-Living-Health. It is hoped the ideas herein will spark different thoughts, shed new lights, and mobilize shifts in points of view.

The work is primarily intended for graduate students at both master's and doctoral levels, as well as for faculty in baccalaureate and higher-degree programs who might find it useful in curriculum development. It is offered as a contribution in the ongoing quest of defining a unique body of nursing knowledge.

Rosemarie Rizzo Parse, Ph.D., R.N.

Acknowledgments

With appreciation to the many predecessors, contemporaries, and successors who continue to coconstitute the evolution of *Man-Living-Health: A Theory of Nursing*. Special thanks and affection go to those people who explicitly lived and participated with the creation of this work and bore witness to its birthing.

- John A. Parse, husband and friend, whose loving presence, limitless support, and fine-honed writing ability immeasureably aided the unfolding of the project.
- Rosella M. Obringer and Frank J. Rizzo, my insightful parents, their children, and their children's children, whose enlivening spirits are always with me.
- Dr. A. Barbara Coyne, friend and colleague, whose engaging presence and profound scholarliness enhanced the evolution of the theory.
- Dr. Mary Jane Smith, friend and colleague, whose high scholarly standards and persistent criticism and meta criticism gave focus to the construction of the theory.
- Mrs. Clara Cuda, whose loyal, precise, and energetic assistance lightened the burden.
- The budding young scholars and graduate students, in whose presence the theory unfolded—week after week—year after year—as we engaged in the teaching-learning process.

- A once and future friend, whose ever present meta perspective of my many unfolding projects illuminated the struggle and the moments of joy all at once.

Rosemarie Rizzo Parse, Ph.D., R.N.

Contents

I. EMERGENCE OF A PARADIGM OF NURSING 1

II. EVOLUTION OF THE THEORY OF MAN-LIVING-HEALTH 9

III. ASSUMPTIONS ABOUT MAN AND HEALTH ROOTED IN THE HUMAN SCIENCES 23

IV. PRINCIPLES, CONCEPTS, AND THEORETICAL STRUCTURES OF MAN-LIVING-HEALTH 37

V. EMPIRICAL ASPECTS OF MAN-LIVING-HEALTH: A THEORY OF NURSING 75

EPILOGUE 173

GLOSSARY 177

BIBLIOGRAPHY 181

INDEX 197

Illustrations

Schema 1 Comparison of Nursing Paradigms 14

Schema 2 Principles, Tenets, and Concepts from Rogers and Existential-Phenomenology 22

Schema 3 Evolution of Assumptions from Principles, Tenets, and Concepts 34

Schema 4 Concept-Assumption Interface 35

Schema 5 Assumptions with Related Concepts 36

Schema 6 Relationship of Principles, Concepts, and Theoretical Structures of Man-Living-Health 69

Schema 7 Evolution of the Theory of Man-Living-Health 70

Schema 8 The Theory of Man-Living-Health 73

Schema 9 Sample Conceptual Framework, Themes, Support Theories, and Theorists 101

Schema 10 Sample Graduate Nursing Program Evaluation Model 152

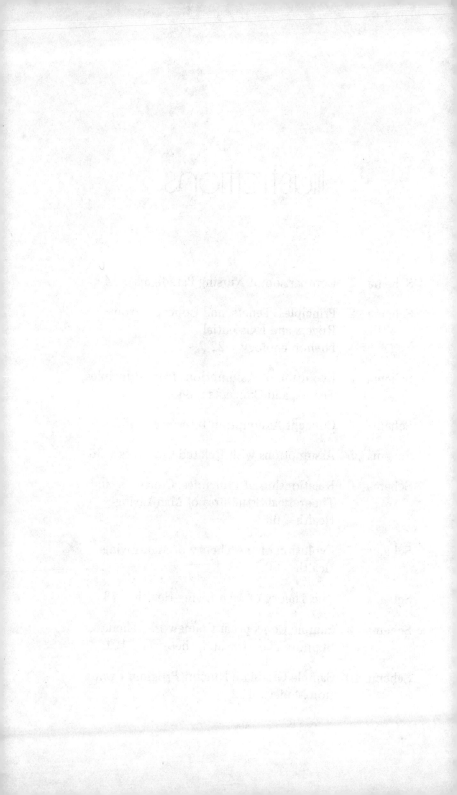

CHAPTER 1

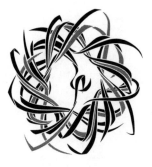

Emergence of a Paradigm of Nursing

■

To posit the idea of nursing rooted in the human
sciences is to make explicit an alternative to the traditional practice of nursing as a medical model grounded
in the natural sciences. Historically, nursing has been a
health profession closely related to medicine in the cure
of human beings, and it is just beginning to justify its
claims as an emerging discipline. There are many vari-
ables related to the fact that nursing has held tena-
ciously to its medical connections and theories. These
include the role of women in history and the power of
organized medicine. Nursing's close association with
medicine has understandably led to its grounding in
the natural sciences. This book proposes a grounding
for nursing in the human sciences. And there is a significant difference between a natural science approach
and a human science approach. The fact that nursing
is currently practiced and taught as a natural science,
medical model is borne out in the literature. Many
nursing textbooks are organized in a format that focuses
on information about disease processes and their effects
on individuals. And, as in other natural sciences, nursing
research and literature have sought mainly to quantify
and to determine specific cause-effect relationships
for use in the practice of nursing. In traditional nursing,
methodologies from the physical sciences historically
have dealt with disease and trauma and their attendant
treatment and cure. "Tasks, technology and teaching
have been the predominant nursing frames of reference
. . . from a reading of the first 25 years of *Nursing
Research*."[1] More specifically, natural science nursing
has, since its inception, dealt with the quantification

[1] Rosemary Ellis, "Fallabilities, Fragments and Frames: Contemplations on 25 years of Research in Medical-Surgical Nursing,"
Nursing Research 26 (3), May-June 1977, p. 181.

of man and his illness rather than the qualification of man's total experience with health. Man has been approached through the study of parts rather than through a study of man as a living unity. Man's participative experience with health situations has been virtually ignored. Nursing, rooted in the human sciences, focuses on man as a living unity and man's qualitative participation with health experiences.

Conceptual approaches to nursing, differing slightly from the traditional, are emerging. These conceptualizations incorporate open and closed systems, total and wholistic views of man, and interactional and transactional relations.[2,3,4] The emergence of a variety of conceptual systems of nursing bears witness to the coming of age of nursing as a discipline. The discipline of nursing is emerging as do all disciplines, through a process of conceptual development, from the prescientific phase to the scientific phase. This began with the institution of formal nursing in the middle of the nineteenth century, when prescientific practice was based on intuitive knowing with an informal structure. Nursing continues to emerge as a discipline with current practice based on conceptual systems having a formalized structure.

This book, *Man-Living-Health: A Theory of Nursing*, is grounded in the human sciences. It synthesizes Martha E. Rogers's principles and concepts about man with major tenets and concepts from existential-phenomenological thought to create an emergent conceptual system. Rogers authored the landmark book, *An Introduction to the Theoretical Basis of*

[2] Imogene King, *Toward a Theory of Nursing* (New York: John Wiley & Sons, 1971).

[3] Josephine Paterson and Loretta T. Zderad, *Humanistic Nursing* (New York: John Wiley & Sons, 1976).

[4] Joan P. Riehl and Callista Roy, *Conceptual Models for Nursing Practice* (New York: Appleton-Century-Crofts, 1980).

Nursing, and created what was and is the first definitive nursing science conceptual framework. A conceptual framework represents "a matrix of concepts which together describe the focus of inquiry."[5] Rogers's work is rooted in Ludwig von Bertalanffy's general system theory and in the works of Teilhard de Chardin, Michael Polanyi, and Kurt Lewin. Søren Kierkegaard, a non-phenomenologist, founded existentialism; Edmund Husserl, who is a non-existentialist, created phenomenology. Kierkegaard and Husserl interface in their view of man as being human and more than atomistic. Martin Heidegger first recognized the congruence of these two authors' thoughts and merged existentialism and phenomenology to create existential-phenomenology. The existential-phenomenological movement, evolved primarily through Heidegger, was promulgated and disseminated widely through the works of Jean-Paul Sartre, Maurice Merleau-Ponty, and others. Rogers, Heidegger, Sartre, and Merleau-Ponty, then, are the predominant theorists drawn upon in the creation of the nursing theory Man-Living-Health.

To draw upon the work of these theorists, of course, is to build upon a solid foundation and to maintain a bridge to the past necessary in the establishment of any scientific theory. It is easy to forget in the process, however, that this foundation is only recently solidified, this bridge only recently completed. Earlier in this century, and even now for Rogers, these various theorists and their works were as much criticized as acclaimed, as much reviled as admired, and as much ignored as followed. Consistent with history dating back to Darwin, Copernicus, and beyond, these plowers of new ground and these creators of new theories found the initial going difficult. Their problems have been partially of their own making. In *The Structure of Scientific Revo-*

---

[5] Margaret Newman, *Theory Development in Nursing* (Philadelphia: F. A. Davis Company, 1979), pp. 5-6.

lutions, Thomas S. Kuhn wrote that, in solving problems or forming a theory, a scientist has two choices. The scientist may attempt to solve the problem within the existing system, as Copernicus could have attempted within the Ptolemaic theory, or create a new system, a counter instance, a revolutionary process. The Darwins, Copernicuses, Kierkegaards, and Rogerses of the world have chosen the latter.

To do so, of course, is to wander in the wilderness, to want for honor, and to lack disciples, at least for a time. Ultimately, and happily, the Copernicuses have their Galileos, the Darwins their Huxleys, and the Kierkegaards their Heideggers. Rogers, too, has her disciples, and she continues to attract more. To follow Rogers, of course, is to forsake the theory of medicine as a paradigm of nursing and to affirm a different conceptual system.

The emergence of a paradigm in any science usually comes about when the scientists of that particular discipline recognize an anomaly between existing theory and the nature of the phenomenon it seeks to describe. Those scientists who stimulate the change, those visionaries who create the new paradigm, view the anomaly as more than just a puzzle. Puzzles, after all, are the historic and daily challenges, the ones that can ultimately be solved within the existing order. Forward-looking scientists instead view this anomaly as a real counter instance, a crisis situation, one requiring a new articulation of the relationships among the phenomena and calling for a different view of the fundamentals. Lavoisier, for example, promulgated such a view when he published his theory on chemical compounds, diverging forever from the elemental earth theory of Priestly and others.

Recognition of an anomaly between the theory of medicine and the nature of nursing is at the center of the emergence of the paradigm for nursing rooted in the human sciences. The theory of medicine is grounded in the view of man as a mechanistic bio-psycho-social being, the sum of parts. Consequently, practice focuses on diagnosis and treatment in curing, controlling, and preventing disease. The nature of nursing is grounded in the view of man as a unified being, more than the sum of parts, and focuses on caring and healing.[6,7] Thus, the phenomenon of nursing has a different root and focus from medicine. This fundamental difference is not viewed as a puzzle to be solved but as a counter instance of the same type and mode of crisis just described. And a crisis of that proportion requires a different fundamental view of the familiar. The nursing paradigm proposed in this book identifies unitary man as one who coparticipates with the environment in creating and becoming, and who is whole, open, and free to choose ways of living health. This is in contradistinction to a paradigm that views man as the sum of parts, acted upon and delimited by such terms as disease and pathology.

The emergence of a new paradigm of nursing grounded in the human sciences is illuminated in the remaining chapters of this book. Rogers's three principles, helicy, complementarity, and resonancy, as well as the emerging concepts about man, energy field, openness, pattern and organization, and four-dimensionality, are explained. The fundamental tenets of existential-phenomenology, human subjectivity, and intentionality, with the emerging ideas of coconstitution, coexistence, and situated freedom, are also discussed.

Assumptions about man and health emerge from a synthesis of these principles, tenets, and concepts. These assumptions are explicated, and the emergent

[6] Madeleine Leininger, "Transcultural Nursing and a Proposed Conceptual Framework," in *Transcultural Nursing Care of Infants and Children*, ed. M. Leininger (Salt Lake City, Utah: University of Utah College of Nursing, 1977).

[7] Virginia Henderson, "The Nature of Nursing," *The American Journal of Nursing* 64 (8), August 1964, pp. 62-68.

principles, concepts, and theoretical structures of Man-Living-Health are explained. Some empirical implications of Man-Living-Health relative to nursing research, practice, and education are discussed. A research methodology to uncover the lived experience of Man-Living-Health is suggested, and a sample curriculum plan for a program leading to a master of science in nursing degree is proposed.

CHAPTER II

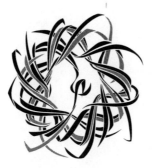

Evolution of
the Theory of
Man-Living-Health

■

MAN-LIVING-HEALTH:
A NURSING PARADIGM

Nursing, as it is practiced and taught in the United States, historically has been viewed as an emerging natural science. This book is an effort to create a paradigm of nursing rooted in the human sciences. There are differences between a natural and a human science approach. A natural science posits methodologies that elicit quantitative data from observable phenomena and reveal causal relationships. Natural sciences deal with the reduction to parts of the phenomena being studied. These parts are examined by using criteria from a predetermined theoretical framework. "The working model of the natural sciences is constituted by the concepts of a causal order in a physical world and their particular methodology consists of procedures for discovering it."[1] The human sciences, on the other hand, posit a methodology directed toward uncovering the meaning of phenomena as humanly experienced. Human science methodology is the study of unitary man's participative experience with a situation. "The human sciences are possible only because we directly participate in their subject matter."[2] The human sciences aim at understanding the connectedness of life itself.[3] The method of inquiry leads to the creation of a theoretical framework and the generation of hypotheses. The theory posited in this book has as a fundamental tenet man's participation

[1] Wilhelm Dilthey, *Pattern and Meaning in History* (New York: Harper & Row, 1961), p. 109.
[2] John Macquarrie, *Martin Heidegger* (Richmond, Virginia: John Knox Press, 1968), p. 36.
[3] Dilthey, *Pattern and Meaning in History*, p. 109.

11

in health. Verification for this theory is expected
through methodologies that uncover the connectedness
of lived experiences.

Nursing has traditionally been taught and practiced as
a medical science. Philosophically, nursing has adopted
the model of man historically employed by medical
science, *homo naturus.* The major idea underpinning
this medical model is a particulate view of man. The
knowledge base is organized into the classical divisions
of medical-surgical, pediatric, obstetric, and psychiatric
nursing, paralleling the medical specialties. A more
recent theoretical approach in nursing posits man as
a bio-psycho-socio-spiritual organism. This approach is
in keeping with the natural science view of man. The
medical model, nearly as far back as Galen, has focused
upon a certain mind-body dichotomy, a Cartesian
dualism that predates Descartes by centuries but still
permeates much of our modern thinking. And this
dualism has been successful in the practice of medicine
as medicine and in the emergence of medical science.
To treat *homo naturus* medically is to deal with bio-
physiological systems in which tissues, organs, and
their various diseases are viewed and treated separately.
Nursing's emergence with medicine in the study of man
created one science, namely, medical science, with the
coparticipation of both medicine and nursing. This
approach seriously curtailed the development of a
unique and distinct body of nursing knowledge, even
though Florence Nightingale set forth a view of man
as more than the sum of parts, a view of nursing as
knowledge distinct from medical knowledge, and a
focus on health rather than illness.[4] In the main, then,
nursing, philosophically and in practice, mirrors the
natural science approach and, with some exceptions,
accepts the medical model. A view of nursing, different
from medicine and yet complementary to medicine,

[4] Florence Nightingale, *Notes on Nursing* (Philadelphia: J. P.
Lippincott Company, 1946), preface.

is possible when it is viewed as rooted in the human sciences.

A theory of nursing rooted in the human sciences is a system of interrelated concepts describing unitary man's interrelating with the environment while co-creating health. Essential to the theory is the man-environment interrelationship, coconstitution of health, the meaning unitary man gives to being and becoming, and man's freedom in each situation to choose alternative ways of becoming.

This theory relates assumptions about man and health that are synthesized into the principles, concepts, and theoretical structures of Man-Living-Health. These assumptions emerge from Rogers's principles and concepts about man and from the existential-phenomenological thought, primarily, of Heidegger, Sartre, and Merleau-Ponty.

Concepts from Rogers's nursing science model correspond to von Bertalanffy's general system theory and are synthesized with concepts from existential-phenomenological thought to create the new paradigm. Schema 1 is a comparison of the nursing paradigm Man-Living-Health and the medical science nursing paradigm relative to a view of man and health and the primary goal of practice.

The next two sections explain the principles and concepts from Rogers and the tenets and concepts from existential-phenomenology that have been synthesized in the creation of the theory of Man-Living-Health.

ROGERS'S PRINCIPLES AND CONCEPTS RELATED TO THE THEORY OF MAN-LIVING-HEALTH

Rogers, in "Nursing: A Science of Unitary Man," posits three major principles of nursing science—helicy, complementarity, and resonancy—and four building

SCHEMA 1. COMPARISON OF NURSING PARADIGMS

	Man-Living-Health Nursing Paradigm	Medical Science Nursing Paradigm
View of Man	Synergistic—more than and different from the sum of parts characterized by patterns of relating	Mechanistic—the sum of parts characterized by bio-psycho-socio-spiritual aspects
	Open being coextensive with universe	Closed system separated from universe
	Mutual simultaneous inter-relationship	Linear causality
	Coconstituting with the environment	Adapting to the environment
	Negentropic	Entropic
	Free to choose in situation	Confined by situation
View of Health	Process of becoming as experienced by a person	Physical, mental, and social state of well-being as defined by norms
Goal	To guide the family in choosing among possibil-ities in the changing health process	To prevent illness and care for the sick in the promotion of health

blocks—energy field, openness, pattern and organization, and four-dimensionality.[5] These are the specific ideas from Rogers used in the creation of the theory of Man-Living-Health. These principles and concepts will be discussed in the next part of this chapter.

Principles

Rogers's three principles are helicy, complementarity, and resonancy.

[5] Martha E. Rogers, "Nursing: A Science of Unitary Man," in *Conceptual Models for Nursing Practice,* eds. Joan P. Riehl and Callista Roy (New York: Appleton-Century-Crofts, 1980).

HELICY

The principle of helicy specifies that "the nature and direction of human and environmental change is continuously innovative, probablistic, and characterized by increasing diversity of human field and environmental field pattern and organization. . ."[6] This principle postulates that man and environment evolve in mutual simultaneous negentropic emergence. It relates to the concepts of energy field and four-dimensionality.

COMPLEMENTARITY

Helicy subsumes the principle of complementarity, which emphasizes that the human and environmental field interaction "is continuous, mutual, and simultaneous."[7]

RESONANCY

The principle of resonancy postulates that "the human field and the environmental field are identified by wave pattern and organization manifesting continuous change from lower-frequency, longer wave patterns to higher-frequency, shorter wave patterns."[8] There is a rhythmical energy interchange between man and environment expressed in wave patterns. This principle relates to the concepts of openness and pattern and organization.

Concepts

The major concepts relating to Rogers's principles are energy field, openness, pattern and organization, and four-dimensionality.

[6] Ibid., p. 333.
[7] Ibid.
[8] Ibid.

ENERGY FIELD

Rogers posits unitary man as an indivisible energy field.[9] She says that the unity of man is a reality.—"Man is a unified whole possessing his own integrity and manifesting characteristics that are more than and different from the sum of his parts."[10] Man transcends the deductions made from the study of chemistry, biology, psychology, and sociology, and cannot be explained by the ideated integration of parts. This idea of man as a unified whole dates back to the ancient Greeks; but with emergent technologies, more and more emphasis was directed toward the study of the segments of man. Yet, man cannot be totalized by an additive process. The human field interacts with the environmental field and, synergistically, man and environment enhance each other.

Polanyi supports the view of man as more than and different from the sum of parts. He says ". . . understanding of a whole appreciates the coherence of its subject matter and thus acknowledges the existence of a value that is absent from the constituent particular."[11] To study unitary man, then, means to study man's wholeness, the characteristics of which emerge through pattern and organization.

OPENNESS

Another concept, openness, refers to man as an open system, an energy field contiguous with the universe. Rogers states that man and environment, mutually and simultaneously, interchange energy.[12] She posits nega-

[9] Ibid., p. 330.

[10] Martha E. Rogers, *An Introduction to the Theoretical Basis of Nursing* (Philadelphia: F. A. Davis Company, 1970), p. 47.

[11] Michael Polanyi, *Personal Knowledge* (Chicago: University of Chicago Press, 1958), p. 327.

[12] Rogers, *Theoretical Basis of Nursing*, pp. 49–54.

tion of man as a closed system, a steady state, and an adaptive organism. Man and environment interrelate in negentropic emergence, which is irreversible movement toward greater diversity and complexity.[13]

PATTERN AND ORGANIZATION

Rogers specifies that man can be recognized through human field pattern and organization.[14] Man and environment change continuously, yet there is continuity in this ever-changing process. The pattern and organization of man and the pattern and organization of environment are rhythmical expressions of unity. These rhythmical expressions are novel, diverse wave patterns.[15] Man's energy field pattern distinguishes him from the environmental energy field.

FOUR-DIMENSIONALITY

The concept of four-dimensionality postulates man and environment as four-dimensional energy fields. These energy fields are in simultaneous, continuous, and mutual interaction and are "characterized by continuously fluctuating imaginary boundaries."[16] Four-dimensionality specifies a world with neither space nor time where the human field is a "relative present."[17] Four-dimensional reality points to man's continuous innovative emergence and sheds light on the meaning of paranormal experiences as evolutionary emergents.

Rogers believes, then, that unitary man is a four-dimensional energy field, recognized by a distinct

[13] Rogers, "Nursing: A Science of Unitary Man," p. 331.
[14] Ibid., p. 331.
[15] Ibid.
[16] Ibid., pp. 333–334.
[17] Ibid.

rhythmical pattern and organization, openly changing negentropically and irreversibly with the four-
dimensional environmental field. Rogers's principles
of helicy, complementarity, and resonancy, and the
concepts of energy field, openness, pattern and organization, and four-dimensionality have been discussed.
These, along with the existential-phenomenological
tenets and concepts, underpin the assumptions about
man and health in the theory of Man-Living-Health.

EXISTENTIAL-PHENOMENOLOGICAL
TENETS AND CONCEPTS

Following are the existential-phenomenological tenets
of intentionality and human subjectivity and the concepts of coexistence, situated freedom, and coconstitution that are synthesized with Rogers's principles and
concepts in the creation of a nursing paradigm rooted
in the human sciences.

Tenets

The existential-phenomenological tenets of human
subjectivity and intentionality evolve from Kierkegaard's belief about man as subject and Husserl's belief
about man as unity with the world.

INTENTIONALITY

The basic tenet, intentionality, posits that man is by
nature an intentional being. This means that in being
human man is open, knows, and is present to the world.
To be man, then, is to be intentional and to be involved
with the world through a fundamental nature of knowing, being present and open.[18] Man is involved with

[18] Martin Heidegger, *Being and Time* (New York: Harper & Row,
1962), pp. 86–87.

the world in creating the self-project of personal becoming. The creating of the self-project emerges from
man's historicity and facticity. Man's historicity reflects
connections with predecessors and contemporaries in
creating the who one is at a given moment, and facticity
is the immediate situation in which man finds self. Man
is in situation as an already present being and a potential
not-yet, open and present to the world. That man
transcends the present bears witness to freedom and
the desire to reach beyond self. This freedom and desire
to reach beyond self relates to intentionality in that
man chooses in situation a stand with the world and, in
so doing, achieves potentials and possibilities all at
once.[19] This tenet gives rise to the concepts of coexistence and situated freedom.

HUMAN SUBJECTIVITY

The basic tenet, human subjectivity, posits that con-
scious man by nature is no-thing but, rather, a unity of
being and non-being. This means that man is more than
a cosmic being or thing;[20] man is a unity of the subject-
world relationship. In subjectivity man encounters the
world and is present to it in a dialectical relationship.[21]
Man grows through this relationship, giving meaning to
the projects that emerge in the process of becoming.
Man coparticipates in the emergence of projects through
choosing to live certain values. This relates to human
subjectivity in that man, by nature, participates with the
world in cocreation of self. This tenet gives rise to the
concept of coconstitution.

Concepts

From the existential-phenomenological tenets of intentionality and human subjectivity emerge these

[19] Ibid., pp. 185–186.
[20] Ibid., p. 73.
[21] Ibid., p. 85.

assumptions about man: man coconstitutes situations with the world, man experiences existence as coexistence, and man has freedom in situation.

COCONSTITUTION

"Man coconstitutes situations" refers to the idea that the meaning emerging in any situation is related to the particular constituents of that situation. Man is enabled and limited by the man-world dialectic through which situations come into being. Man interrelates with the various views of the world and others and indeed cocreates these views by a personal presence.[22] Man by nature is present to the world and, all at once, open to possibilities and, as such, participates in the creation of the world.[23]

COEXISTENCE

"Man experiences existence as coexistence" means that man is not alone in any dimension of becoming. Man, an emerging being, is in the world with others; indeed, even the act of coming into the world is through others. Man knows self in the comprehension of dispersed concrete achievements and through the perceptions of others. Without others one would not know that one is. To exist, then, is to coexist as the possibility of transcending self to be more than one is at a given point in space-time.[24]

SITUATED FREEDOM

"Man has freedom in situation" means that, reflectively and prereflectively, one participates in choosing the

[22] Maurice Merleau-Ponty, *Phenomenology of Perception* (New York: Humanities Press, 1974), pp. 369–409.

[23] Heidegger, *Being and Time*, pp. 252–417.

[24] Merleau-Ponty, *Phenomenology of Perception*, pp. 346–365.

situations in which one finds oneself as well as one's attitude toward the situations. That is, how a particular situation emerges is related to man's facticity and to earlier choosings, both those reflected upon and those participated in without prior reflection. Man's facticity is that which man was born to. The givens in situations, then, are present from earlier choosings and from man's facticity, and the emergent possibilities are enabled and limited by these givens. Man is a being who can remember past experiences as past events. One creates a personal remembrance by choosing the order and arrangement of reflections on these past events as one gives meaning to situations. In choosing ways of being with situations, one expresses value priorities. Man is compelled to take a stand toward the emergent desires and feelings evolving in situations. One always chooses; as Sartre says, even ". . . not to choose is in fact to choose not to choose. . . ."[25] Choices are made without full knowledge of the outcomes yet with full responsibility for the consequences.

The principles and concepts from Rogers and the tenets and concepts from existential-phenomenological thought used in the creation of the theory of Man-Living-Health have been presented. Schema 2 depicts these principles, tenets, and concepts.

[25] Jean-Paul Sartre, *Being and Nothingness* (New York: Washington Square Press, 1966), p. 619.

SCHEMA 2. PRINCIPLES, TENETS, AND CONCEPTS FROM ROGERS AND EXISTENTIAL-PHENOMENOLOGY

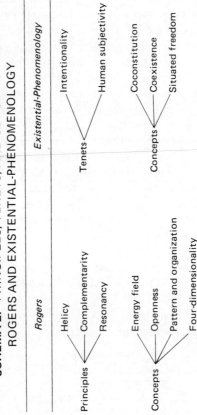

Rogers	Existential-Phenomenology
Principles — Helicy, Complementarity, Resonancy	Tenets — Intentionality, Human subjectivity
Concepts — Energy field, Openness, Pattern and organization, Four-dimensionality	Concepts — Coconstitution, Coexistence, Situated freedom

CHAPTER III

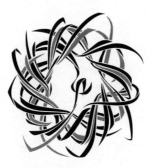

Assumptions About
Man and Health
Rooted in
the Human Sciences

■

The principles, tenets, and concepts described in Chapter II from Rogers, Heidegger, Merleau-Ponty, and Sartre are synthesized in the creation of the assumptions about man and health, underpinning a view of nursing grounded in the human sciences.

These assumptions are

- Man is coexisting while coconstituting rhythmical patterns with the environment.
- Man is an open being, freely choosing meaning in situation, bearing responsibility for decisions.
- Man is a living unity continuously coconstituting patterns of relating.
- Man is transcending multidimensionally with the possibles.
- Health is an open process of becoming, experienced by man.
- Health is a rhythmically coconstituting process of the man-environment interrelationship.
- Health is man's patterns of relating value priorities.
- Health is an intersubjective process of transcending with the possibles.
- Health is unitary man's negentropic unfolding.

A discussion of these assumptions follows. Each assumption connects three specific concepts in a unique way. Each of the seven concepts discussed in Chapter II—energy field, openness, pattern and organization, four-dimensionality, coconstitution, coexistence, and situated freedom—is related at least once with each of the others in the creation of the assumptions. Some concepts appear in more assumptions than others. The unique interrelationship of the three concepts in each

assumption confirms each as essential to the underpinning of the theory of Man-Living-Health.

ASSUMPTION 1: MAN IS COEXISTING
WHILE COCONSTITUTING
RHYTHMICAL PATTERNS
WITH THE ENVIRONMENT

Assumption 1 synthesizes the concepts of coexistence,
coconstitution, and pattern and organization. The
assumption means that man exists with others, evolving
simultaneously and in cadence with the environment.
Man, a recognizable pattern in the man-environment
interrelationship, unfolds with contemporaries the
ideas of predecessors. This interrelationship is the
continuity that connects past with future, bearing
witness to man's coexistence with all men. To say that
man coexists means that man lives all at once with
ancestors, successors, and contemporaries through
personal interrelationships, ideas, and future planning.
That man coexists in a situation is evidence of his
participation in coconstituting it. Man coparticipates
with the environment in simultaneously evolving the
individual patterns of relating that distinguish an individual from the environmental pattern and the generic
pattern of man. Patterns of relating are created through
the mutual rhythmical man-environment energy interchange and reflect the wholeness of both man and
environment. Man, then, is a pattern of patterns of
relating. Man as pattern and organization is distinct
from the pattern and organization of environment.
Patterns of relating are the individual's unique way of
being recognized. Man, coexisting with environment,
coconstitutes rhythmical patterns of relating.

ASSUMPTION 2: MAN IS AN OPEN BEING, FREELY CHOOSING MEANING IN SITUATION, BEARING RESPONSIBILITY FOR DECISIONS

Assumption 2 synthesizes the concepts of situated freedom, openness, and energy field. It means that man in open energy interchange with the environment chooses ways of being in situation and is accountable for the choices. Synergistic man, unique among beings in the universe, feels with the environment. Man appreciates art, music, and moments of joy and is touched by birthings and dyings, which are the rhythmical happenings in day-to-day living. These happenings are created as man chooses the meanings of a situation and, through this choosing, the possibilities that man can become. Choosing meaning points to the birthings and dyings inherent in each decision. This means that, in choosing one thing, man gives up another and in this way is both enabled and limited. Man incarnates lived paradox just as being, all at once, bears witness to nonbeing. Non-being, as a complex phenomenon, can be explained as inherent in being itself. It is more than being. The presence of man with the world is the being itself that surfaces the fact of non-being, that is, being dead or meaningless. Man is aware of the possibility of loss of self through dying, and he sees the potential of being cut off from the possibility of affirming self. Possibilities for man are relational in that man and environment coparticipate in their emergence. This emergence is through energy interchange and toward greater complexity. Man and environment, then, interchange energy to create what is in the world, and man chooses the meaning given to the situations he cocreates. Man is responsible for all outcomes of choices even though he does not know them when making a decision.

ASSUMPTION 3: MAN IS A
LIVING UNITY CONTINUOUSLY
COCONSTITUTING PATTERNS
OF RELATING

Assumption 3 synthesizes the concepts of energy field, pattern and organization, and coconstitution. Man is synergistic, more than and different from the sum of parts, and is recognized through the ways of being, cocreated with environment. Man as more than and different from the sum of parts means that man cannot be divided into psychological, biological, and sociological components. Man, unified, can be recognized through individual patterns of relating. These are not particulate but ever-changing as man coconstitutes his becoming. Man's patterns of relating are cocreated in the energy interchange that occurs between man and environment. As energy is interchanged, the pattern and organization of man unfolds images that reflect man's wholeness. These images are the unique, ordered patterns of relating that are changing in nature and distinguish one human being from another. Coconstituted patterns of relating are unitary man's ways of being and are illuminated through gesture, movement, gaze, posture, touch, and speech.

ASSUMPTION 4: MAN
IS TRANSCENDING
MULTIDIMENSIONALLY
WITH THE POSSIBLES

Assumption 4 synthesizes specifically the concepts of four-dimensionality, situated freedom, and openness. This assumption means that there is a mutual energy interchange between man and environment as man chooses to move beyond the actual, the contextual situation, toward possibilities. This movement is not repeatable, and it is irreversible. Man, in open inter-relationship, experiences multidimensionally; that is, the man-environment energy interchange occurs simultaneously and relatively at many universe levels. Space and time are unified multidimensional entities, unbounded and nonsequential. There is no absolute space or absolute time in relation to events. Space-time is interrelated with events simultaneously. The whole structure of space-time is related to the flow of probability patterns of interconnections of all that is in the universe. Space-time is a unity of rhythmically flowing interconnected wave patterns. These are the webs of interconnections of the man-environment interrelationship and are the various universes that man lives reflectively and prereflectively all at once. These webs of interconnections are complementary and synergistic. Complementarity implies a unity of apparent opposites; that is, the positive coexists simultaneously with the negative, life with non-life, up with down. Synergy implies the maximization of coexistent energies, emerging together to create possibilities with the various universes lived simultaneously. In the man-environment interrelationship, man chooses from the many options available in multidimensional experiences. One exceeds who one is through mutual and simultaneous energy interchange while imaging other possibilities. The imaged possibilities go beyond space-time boundaries and surface options from which man chooses in becoming. These choices are the new actuals, the contextual situations in relative space-time boundaries. The experience of events, then, is related to the relative perspective of the one experiencing them. The new actuals illuminate other possibilities, and man reaches toward them while continually becoming more complex and more diverse through choosing. This is the process of transcending with the possibles.

ASSUMPTION 5: HEALTH IS AN
OPEN PROCESS OF BECOMING,
EXPERIENCED BY MAN

Assumption 5 synthesizes the concepts of openness, situated freedom, and coconstitution. This assumption means that, in the interrelational movement between man and environment, there is a continuous negentropic interchange of energy that both enables and limits becoming. Becoming is man's continuous growing through energy interchange with the environment toward the not-yet that is more diverse and more complex. Inherent in growing is choosing who one will be in situation. Choosing is from a unique perspective that is angular, relative, and single-sided though coconstituted with others. That is, man's view of the options is from the history man has been becoming. An experience of a situation, while cocreated with others, belongs to one human being only. Choosing some options, by nature, eliminates others so that possibilities are cocreated and experienced perspectively in the process of becoming, living health. Living health, then, is an incarnation of man's choosings. It is experienced multidimensionally and lived uniquely but described as relatively sequenced in time, ordered in space, and shared through energy. The unique perspective of each human being experiencing self in the man-environment energy interchange is health.

ASSUMPTION 6: HEALTH
IS A RHYTHMICALLY
COCONSTITUTING PROCESS
OF THE MAN-ENVIRONMENT
INTERRELATIONSHIP

The concepts synthesized in Assumption 6 are coconstitution, pattern and organization, and four-dimensionality. This assumption means that health, man's becoming, is an undulating energy interchange cocreated as man and environment interrelate. Becoming is man's continuous carving out, in cadence with the environment, recognizable patterns of relating. The carving out involves one's changing from what one is to what one wants to be. Changing is an ongoing pulselike rhythm, an ebb and flow of connecting-separating and emerging anew. The connecting-separating phenomenon is complementary and simultaneous. This means that in each connecting there already is a separating. The separation is from that which man is not dwelling with at the moment. It is this man-environment connecting and separating that coconstitutes the emergence of man's health as a relative present. Man, though, always moving simultaneously with the environment, flows closely with certain phenomena and distant from others. Man is multidimensionally connecting and separating all at once. In this connecting, man dwells with a particular situation and, through energy interchange, new ways of being emerge unique to that coming together. Man's health, then, is this rhythmic process of changing through the simultaneous connecting and separating of man with environment.

ASSUMPTION 7: HEALTH IS MAN'S PATTERNS OF RELATING VALUE PRIORITIES

Assumption 7 synthesizes the concepts of situated freedom, pattern and organization, and openness. This assumption means that health is man's style of living chosen cherished ideals. Health is a synthesis of man's values selected from multidimensional experiences cocreated in open energy interchange with environment. Man makes choices from options affirming as cherished certain ways of being. These ways of being emerge in recognizable patterns and reflect man's priorities and increasing complexity. These patterns of relating are man's way of languaging values. They are everchanging as man continually appropriates new values synergistically. The new values incarnated in day-to-day living emerge as diverse changing priorities. The patterns of relating value priorities constitute man's health.

ASSUMPTION 8: HEALTH IS AN INTERSUBJECTIVE PROCESS OF TRANSCENDING WITH THE POSSIBLES

Assumption 8 synthesizes the concepts of openness, situated freedom, and coexistence. It means that health is reaching beyond the actual to the possible through subject-to-subject energy interchange, an interchange that occurs between man and man and between man and other environmental phenomena. The essence of subject-to-subject experience originates in coexistence with others and is man's genuine presence with the interrelational. This genuine presence calls forth a risking of self and a confronting of the other. The risking of self is illuminated through the rhythm of revealing-concealing and reflects man's choosing ways of becoming more complex and more diverse. It means giving up the familiar to struggle with the unfamiliar toward an imaged not-yet as one, all at once, reveals and conceals who one is and can become. Man's risking of self occurs in concert with the confronting of the other, a synergistic rhythm that propels both toward more complex possibilities. The rhythm reveals itself in patterns of struggling and leaping beyond. Health is this continuous intersubjective process of transcending with the possibles.

ASSUMPTION 9: HEALTH IS UNITARY MAN'S NEGENTROPIC UNFOLDING

The concepts specifically synthesized in this assumption are energy field, coexistence, and four-dimensionality. This assumption means that health is man synergistically becoming more complex and more diverse in coexistence with others. More specifically, man with others continuously interchanges energy and evolves to a higher order of organization. The idea of man moving toward greater complexity and diversity posits health as a nonspecific entity, continuously transforming as man grows older. Synergistic man's multidimensional experience of coexistence powers and compounds the creation of individual patterns of relating that are revealed as rhythms of Man-Living-Health. Diversity and complexity increase with aging so that at any given moment man as relative present is more than and different from before. This means that space-time-energy events are not repeatable and are irreversibly integrated with individual patterns of relating. Health is the emergent process of man with others unfolding toward greater complexity.

The preceding nine assumptions about man and health were synthesized from the principles, tenets, and concepts of Rogers, Heidegger, Sartre, and Merleau-Ponty. Schema 3 depicts this relationship.

Each assumption connects three specific concepts in a unique way. Each of the seven concepts explained in Chapter II (energy field, openness, pattern and organization, four-dimensionality, coconstitution, coexistence, and situated freedom) is related at least once with each of the others in the creation of the foundational assumptions of the theory of Man-Living-Health. Schema 4 depicts the concepts with the assumptions in which they appear. Schema 5 shows each assumption with the related concepts.

SCHEMA 3. EVOLUTION OF ASSUMPTIONS FROM PRINCIPLES, TENETS, AND CONCEPTS

	Rogers		*Existential-Phenomenology*
Principles	Helicy	*Tenets*	Intentionality
	Complementarity		Human subjectivity
	Resonancy		
Concepts	Energy field	*Concepts*	Coconstitution
	Openness		Coexistence
	Pattern and organization		Situated freedom
	Four-dimensionality		

Assumptions of Man-Living-Health

1. Man is coexisting while coconstituting rhythmical patterns with the environment.
2. Man is an open being, freely choosing meaning in situation, bearing responsibility for decisions.
3. Man is a living unity continuously coconstituting patterns of relating.
4. Man is transcending multidimensionally with the possibles.

5. Health is an open process of becoming, experienced by man.
6. Health is a rhythmically coconstituting process of the man-environment interrelationship.
7. Health is man's patterns of relating value priorities.
8. Health is an intersubjective process of transcending with the possibles.

9. Health is unitary man's negentropic unfolding.

34

SCHEMA 4. CONCEPT-ASSUMPTION INTERFACE

Energy Field	Openness	Pattern and Organization	Four-Dimensionality	Coconstitution	Coexistence	Situated Freedom
Assumptions	Assumptions	Assumptions	Assumptions	Assumptions	Assumptions	Assumptions
2	2	1	4	1	1	2
3	4	3	6	3	8	4
9	5	6	9	5	9	5
	7	7		6		7
	8					8

35

SCHEMA 5.   ASSUMPTIONS WITH RELATED CONCEPTS

1. Man is coexisting while coconstituting rhythmical patterns with the environment.
   - Coconstitution
   - Coexistence
   - Pattern and organization

2. Man is an open being, freely choosing meaning in situation, bearing responsibility for decisions.
   - Situated freedom
   - Openness
   - Energy field

3. Man is a living unity continuously coconstituting patterns of relating.
   - Energy field
   - Coconstitution
   - Pattern and organization

4. Man is transcending multidimensionally with the possibles.
   - Four-dimensionality
   - Situated freedom
   - Openness

5. Health is an open process of becoming, experienced by man.
   - Openness
   - Coconstitution
   - Situated freedom

6. Health is a rhythmically coconstituting process of the man-environment interrelationship.
   - Coconstitution
   - Pattern and organization
   - Four-dimensionality

7. Health is man's patterns of relating value priorities.
   - Pattern and organization
   - Openness
   - Situated freedom

8. Health is an intersubjective process of transcending with the possibles.
   - Coexistence
   - Openness
   - Situated freedom

9. Health is unitary man's negentropic unfolding.
   - Coexistence
   - Energy field
   - Four-dimensionality

CHAPTER IV

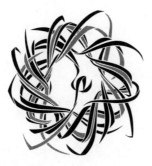

Principles, Concepts, and Theoretical Structures of Man-Living-Health

The assumptions about man and health posited as foundational to this theory of nursing rooted in the human sciences were explained in Chapter III. Man is postulated as a unitary being simultaneously and mutually cocreating with environment rhythmical patterns of relating. As an open being, man freely chooses meaning in situation and bears responsibility for the choices. Man transcends with possibles in negentropically unfolding health.

Man-Living-Health as a theory of nursing emerges from the assumptions. The structuring of the words Man-Living-Health with the hyphen demonstrates a conceptual bond among the words that creates a unity of meaning different from the individual words as they stand alone. The meaning unfolding from this hyphenated structure of man and health points to man's health as ongoing participation with the world. Man-Living-Health is a unitary phenomenon that refers to man's becoming through cocreating rhythmical patterns of relating in open energy interchange with the environment. Man's health, then, is not a linear entity that can be interrupted or qualified by terms such as good, bad, more, or less. It is not man adapting to or coping with environment. Such a description of health dichotomizes and denies man's unitary nature. Unitary man's health is a synthesis of values, a way of living. Goldstein describes health as a value chosen by man. He believes that this value is a characteristic of the true being of man; in fact, it is man's being that is reflective of an interrelationship with the world.[1] Dubos

[1] Kurt Goldstein, "Health as Value," in *New Knowledge in Human Values*, ed. A. H. Maslow (Chicago: Henry Regnery Company, 1959), p. 187.

supports the idea that values and attitudes are related to man's health and that health itself transcends cause-effect relationships.[2] Consistent with this idea is Frankl's belief that health as a value emerges as man structures meaning in situation.[3] Man in energy interchange with the environment continually structures meaning through choosing becoming. This points to Man-Living-Health as a process. Dubos says health is "not a state but a potentiality. . . ."[4] This is congruent with van Kaam's view of the whole of human development.He says, "As man I am both "potentiality" and "emergence" . . . I experience my potentiality as a dynamic tendency toward self emergence. I am not only what I actually am; I am also a constant movement towards self emergence. . . . I am "becoming." I am the potentiality of dying to my life at any moment and to being born to what I am not yet. . . ."[5] Consistent with this view is Ferguson's recent suggestion of an emergent paradigm of man's health, the assumptions of which include health as a view of the whole person with an emphasis on human values and caring.[6] Health, then, from the perspective of this theory of nursing

[2] René Dubos, "Medicine Evolving," in *Ways of Health,* ed. D. S. Sobel (New York: Harcourt Brace Jovanovich, 1979), pp. 42-43.

[3] Viktor E. Frankl, "Significance of the Meaning of Health," in *Religion and Medicine: Essays on Meaning, Valuing and Health,* ed. D. R. Belgium (Ames, Iowa: Iowa State University Press, 1967), pp. 177-185.

[4] René Dubos, "Human Ecology," in *Ways of Health,* ed. D. S. Sobel (New York: Harcourt Brace Jovanovich, 1979) p. 395.

[5] Adrian van Kaam, "Existential Crisis and Human Development," *Humanitas* 10 (2), May 1974, pp. 109-110.

[6] Marilyn Ferguson, *The Aquarian Conspiracy: Personal and Social Transformation in the 1980's* (Los Angeles: J. P. Tarcher, 1980), pp. 246-247.

rooted in the human sciences, is not the opposite of disease or a state that man has but, rather, a continuously changing process that man participates in cocreating. Disease from this perspective is not something a person contracts but rather a pattern of man's interrelationship with the world. Patterns of Man-Living-Health are recognized through the languaging of cocreated relationships that emerge in transcending with the imagined and valued possibles. Man-Living-Health as a unitary phenomenon expresses how man relates with the world through revealing-concealing, enabling-limiting, and connecting-separating. These relationships are rhythmical processes of Man-Living-Health. Through structuring meaning man freely chooses, in situation, ways of originating in unfolding with the possibles. Unfolding with the possibles is powering ways of transforming toward greater complexity. It is incarnating chosen values from options available in multidimensional experiences. Man-Living-Health, then is structuring meaning multidimensionally in cocreating rhythmical patterns of relating while cotranscending with the possibles. The specific principles of the theory of Man-Living-Health are structuring meaning multidimensionally, cocreating rhythmical patterns of relating, and cotranscending with the possibles.

- *Structuring meaning multidimensionally* is cocreating reality through the languaging of valuing and imaging.
- *Cocreating rhythmical patterns of relating* is living the paradoxical unity of revealing-concealing and enabling-limiting while connecting-separating.
- *Cotranscending with the possibles* is powering unique ways of originating in the process of transforming.

Each of these principles is described separately.

PRINCIPLE 1: STRUCTURING MEANING MULTIDIMENSIONALLY IS COCREATING REALITY THROUGH THE LANGUAGING OF VALUING AND IMAGING

Structuring meaning multidimensionally means that Man-Living-Health is continually cocreating reality through assigning meaning to multidimensional experiences that occur all at once. For each person an infinite number of universes exists simultaneously. Reality is a harmony of the many universes made concrete through a person's choices.[7] In the man-environment interrelationship, one chooses from the many options simultaneously available in multidimensional experiences as one originates a worldview and constructs a personal reality. This personal reality incarnates all that a person is, has been, and will become all at once.[8] Constructing reality is giving meaning to unique experience.[9] The unique experience is the individual's perspective incarnated through the personal languaging of imaging and valuing. Imaging, valuing, and languaging, the concepts related to structuring meaning multidimensionally, will be discussed separately.

Imaging

Imaging, the first concept of structuring meaning multidimensionally, is the cocreating of reality that, by its very nature, structures the meaning of an experience. Reality is constructed through man's simultaneous

[7] Bob Toben, *Space-Time and Beyond* (New York: E. P. Dutton, 1975), pp. 25–26.

[8] Wilhelm Dilthey, *Pattern and Meaning in History* (New York: Harper & Row, 1961), pp. 98–99.

[9] Toben, *Space-Time and Beyond*, p. 21.

reflective-prereflective imaging. Reflective-prereflective imaging is the shaping of personal knowledge, the creating of reality explicitly and tacitly all at once. Explicit knowing is articulated logically and reflected upon critically. It has form and substance. Tacit knowing is prearticulate and acritical, "the unreasoned conclusions of our senses."[10] It is quiet and vague and lies hidden from reflective awareness, somewhat anonymous. Man is by nature a questioning being. All that one images is an answer to a question, and the questioning itself is a searching for certainty. "Knowing—that is, picturing [imaging] 'the world' to ourselves is not a purely intellectual affair. . . . our active attitude makes a difference. . . . There are no pure events for us—no 'facts' uncontaminated by the influence of our knowing activities; there are only events colored by and situated in the context of our previously accepted ideas-feeling-beliefs-behavior."[11] Explicit and tacit knowing evolves simultaneously and mutually in man's day-to-day living of reality. This process of coming to know is through indwelling as man integrates the subsidiary awareness of particulars with the focal awareness of wholes, thus unfolding the meanings of experiences.[12] Indwelling is the explicit-tacit process of "utilization of a framework for unfolding our understanding in accordance with the indications and standards imposed by the framework."[13] It is a process of assimilating new ideas into a worldview. For example, one confronted for the first time with the notion that man is

[10] Michael Polanyi, *The Study of Man* (Chicago: University of Chicago Press, 1959), p. 17.

[11] Beatrice Bruteau, *The Psychic Grid* (Wheaton, Illinois: Theosophical Publishing House, 1979), p. 35.

[12] Michael Polanyi, *Knowing and Being* (Chicago: University of Chicago Press, 1969), p. 134.

[13] Ibid.

more than and different from the sum of parts examines
the idea in light of a personal worldview, which is that
man is the sum of parts. One compares the new with
the standards of one's own framework to see whether
or not the idea is compatible. If the idea is compatible,
the person may add the idea to the repertoire of knowledge, expanding horizons of personal knowing. If it is
not, the person may disregard the notion or, if con-
vinced that the idea is supportable, may alter the
standards of the framework to include this idea. This
process of indwelling is how man structures meaning
by cocreating reality. Schutz wrote "the meaning of
our experiences . . . constitutes reality."[14] Greene says
that "To talk of meaning is to talk of interpretation. . . It
is to allow for the fact that there are multiple realities
available to human consciousness and a network of
relationships to effect that have much to do with the
living self."[15] Greene further says that "the province
of science, art, play or dream—is composed of a sect
of more or less compatible experiences. . . . [and always]
. . . interpreted in accord with a characteristic cognitive
style."[16] The significance one gives to an event, then,
is reflective of the whole person.[17] This means that
one structures meanings compatible with one's worldview, which both enables and limits interrogation of
phenomena and the seeking of truth. Imaging reality,
that is, making concrete the meaning of multidimensional experiences, then, incarnates the simultaneity
of the explicit-implicit knowing and is an essential
feature of Man-Living-Health.

[14] Albert Schutz, "On Multiple Realities," in *The Problem of
Social Reality*, Collected Papers, vol. I, ed. Maurice Natanson
(The Hague: Martinue Nijhoff, 1967), pp. 209-212.

[15] Maxine Greene, *Landscapes of Learning* (New York: Teachers
College Press, 1978), p. 16.

[16] Ibid.

[17] Dilthey, *Pattern and Meaning in History*, p. 74.

Valuing

Valuing as the second concept of structuring meaning multidimensionally emerges from the man-environment interchange. It is man's process of confirming cherished beliefs and is reflective of one's world-view. This confirming of beliefs is choosing from imaged options and owning the choices. The choosings are integrated into one's value system, which is a matrix of principles and ideas that guide one's life. The matrix is the framework through which is screened all that is imaged from one's multidimensional experiences.

According to Raths et al. there are seven essentials in the valuing process. An attitude or belief becomes a value for a person when these seven essentials are present. These are choosing freely, choosing from alternatives, reflectively choosing, prizing and cherishing, affirming, acting upon choices, and repeating. The three key activities in the valuing process, then, are *choosing, prizing,* and *acting.*[18] Hall concurs with Raths et al. when he says "to value is to make a choice and act upon it. The choices and acts of one constitute one's history. But as one chooses and acts on values, one also seeks meaning—meaning making and valuing are for all intents and purposes aspects of the same reality."[19] Hall further states that "the act of valuing is the stance the self takes toward the environment such that the self acquires meaning, and the creative development of both the self and the environment is enhanced."[20]

Creating reality, then, is giving meaning to multi-

[18] Louis E. Raths, Merrill Harmin, and Sidney B. Simon, *Values and Teaching* (Columbus, Ohio: Charles E. Merrill, 1978), pp. 27–28.

[19] Brian P. Hall, *The Development of Consciousness: A Confluent Theory of Values* (New York: Paulist Press, 1976), p. 3.

[20] Ibid., p. 26.

dimensional experiences through valuing. A value is a symbol that signifies meaning. For example, a couple adopts a child. This action reflects a prizing of sharing their lives with children. This value was chosen from options available in their multidimensional experiences. The living of this value structures the meaning of family for the couple. Another example is a person changing food-intake patterns to reduce weight in order to present a lean, attractive appearance. This action reflects a prizing, obviously, for presenting a lean, attractive appearance and is a value chosen from options in the person's multidimensional experiences. In these examples, the couple valued having children more than living alone together, and the person valued an attractive lean look more than eating in excess. Both of these values reflect choosing, prizing, and acting upon beliefs. Appropriating a new value is struggling with a decision to affirm a cherished belief; it is choosing one while simultaneously giving up others. In this way, one is both enabled and limited by one's valuing. Through the valuing process, new values are continuously being appropriated and integrated with those held as cherished. The ever-changing values reflect a person's move toward greater complexity. A synthesis of values is one's health. Through choosing valued images from multidimensional experiences, man structures meaning as a feature of Man-Living-Health.

Languaging

Languaging, the third concept of structuring meaning multidimensionally, is expressing valued images. This means that the cocreated images one chooses as values give unique meaning to multidimensional experiences and are symbolized through languaging. One's way of languaging emerges through the man-environment interrelationship and is specifically related to cultural heritage. Languaging is one's representationing of one's structuring of reality[21,22] and is reflective of the interconnectedness of man from generation to generation.[23] People in close association who have common ties and interests cocreate and perpetuate language patterns; thus, while unique realities are structured by each individual, these are cocreated through interrelatedness with others. It is through the process of languaging that each individual symbolizes unique realities. This symbolizing surfaces in the process of speaking and moving. Speaking is "vocal actualization of the tendency to see realities symbolically. . . ."[24] "Moving, like speaking, is a sign or symbol expressing meaning."[25] Symbols are constructed as modes of sharing meaning with others.[26] The meaning expressed is one's worldview and is shared through one's patterns of relating the symbols of words through tonality, tempo, and volume, as well as gesture, gaze, touch, and posture.[27] These symbols are lived all at once in the process of human interchange. When one person encounters another person, rhythmical patterns of relating unfold as words become sentences and are shared with a certain volume at a particular tempo with unique intonation,

[21] Richard Bandler and John Grinder, *The Structure of Magic I* (Palo Alto, California: Science and Behavior Books, 1975), p. 37.

[22] Paul Watzlawick, *The Language of Change* (New York: Basic Books, 1978), p. 16.

[23] Edward T. Hall, *Beyond Culture* (Garden City, New York: Doubleday Anchor Books, 1976), p. 77.

[24] Edward Sapir, *Culture, Language and Personality* (Berkeley and Los Angeles, California: University of California Press, 1966), p. 15.

[25] Ibid., p. 72.

[26] Susanne K. Langer, *Philosophy in a New Key* (Cambridge, Massachusetts: Harvard University Press, 1976), p. 94.

[27] Ludwig von Bertalanffy, "Human Values in a Changing World," in *New Knowledge in Human Values*, ed. A. H. Maslow (Chicago: Henry Regnery Company, 1959), p. 68.

simultaneously with a certain gaze, gesture, touch, and posture. Languaging is not just the content of what a person says with words but how the whole message is revealed in the context of the situation. It is the rhythmical moments of silence, the choice of words and syntax, the intonation, the facial expressions, the gestures, the posture, and that which is not said that constitute the symbolic expression which is characteristic of languaging as a concept of structuring meaning multidimensionally. Languaging is "the intention to unveil the thing itself and go beyond what is said [through speaking and moving] to what what is said signifies."[28] The signification, that is the meaning, is related to choosing the content and structure of the sentences[29] as well as choosing the gestures, intonations, facial expressions, and silences. Themes emerge in the interchange among individuals. The interchange unfolds personal projects and makes concrete valued images. The meanings that surface all at once in a given interchange emerge from the intent and history of the individuals, coconstituting the situation and the context of the situation itself. Each individual participating in an interchange is languaging unique imaged values and is sharing with others a worldview that is the incarnation of one's own history and one's own intention in cocreating the context of the event. Worldview or "world image is the most comprehensive, most complex synthesis of myriads of experiences . . . the . . . ascription of value and meaning . . . a pattern of patterns."[30] In the rhythm of human interchange, an individual both reveals and conceals at once a worldview. No one can reveal all there is about self to the other. The message the other receives is all at once yet not complete. "The

[28] Maurice Merleau-Ponty, *The Prose of the World* (Evanston, Illinois: Northwestern University Press, 1973), p. 102.

[29] Erwin W. Straus, "Sounds, Words, Sentences," in *Language and Language Disturbance*, ed. E. W. Straus (New York: Humanities Press, 1974), p. 101.

[30] Watzlawick, *The Language of Change*, p. 43.

map is not the territory."[31] This means that no individual, the whole territory, can fully understand another; each experiences the other from his own perspective,[32] the map of the other, bearing witness to the ambiguity and mystery that are always present in human encounter. The sharing of worldviews is a complex process in that each individual experiences from a unique perspective and this perspective is never the same as it is for the others present with the same event. Perspective or worldview is not embedded in the context of the situation but rather emerges simultaneously with the choosing of imaged values in the process of human interchange. "What man chooses is what gives structure and meaning to his world."[33] For example, individuals experiencing a given event describe the details of the event differently, though there may be common themes in the description. The differences are related to the unique imaging of values as languaged by each person. Languaging imaged values is creating reality in the process of structuring meaning and is a recognizable feature of Man-Living-Health.

Weaving a "fabric of meaning"[34] in one's life, then, is structuring meaning multidimensionally through imaging, valuing, and languaging. Meaning is continuously changing as the individual is growing more diverse and more complex, as different images give rise to possibilities for new values and original languaging. Structuring meaning multidimensionally is seen in everyday life experiences as an identifiable characteristic of Man-Living-Health. An example of structuring meaning multidimensionally follows.

Bill and Mary decided to get married, creating the

[31] John Grinder and Richard Bandler, *Structure of Magic II* (Palo Alto, California: Science and Behavior Books, 1976), p. 4.

[32] Hall, *Beyond Culture*, p. 69.

[33] Ibid., p. 88.

[34] Langer, *Philosophy in a New Key*, p. 266.

Abrams family. Both Bill and Mary had *imaged* many possibilities for themselves before making the decision. One example is that Mary's family heritage was quite different from Bill's. She had few opportunities to continue her education, and making money was highly *valued* by her parents. Bill's family, on the other hand, of different ethnic background, placed great significance on status and education. Bill's family was unhappy with his choice of Mary as a bride. Both Bill and Mary shared their families' *values* somewhat; but, in sharing each other's worldviews on many issues, they imaged other ways of being together and chose the *valuing* of each other in a marital relationship. Each, through indwelling and assimilating some of the other's worldviews, added new knowledge and cocreated the reality of Mr. and Mrs. Abrams. They chose from alternatives, prized each other, and acted upon the chosen alternative. They *languaged* through symbols such as wedding rings, living together, and a wedding announcement, making concrete their imaged values for each other. The structuring of meaning multidimensionally is exemplified in the decision of Bill and Mary to create the Abrams family, and this is a reflection of Man-Living-Health.

PRINCIPLE 2: COCREATING RHYTHMICAL PATTERNS OF RELATING IS LIVING THE PARADOXICAL UNITY OF REVEALING-CONCEALING AND ENABLING-LIMITING WHILE CONNECTING-SEPARATING

Cocreating rhythmical patterns of relating means that with Man-Living-Health there is an unfolding cadence of coconstituting ways of being with the world. These ways of being are lived rhythmically and are recognized in the man-environment energy interchange in which patterns of Man-Living-Health are identifiable. Rhythmicity is reflected as man and environment move toward shorter, higher-frequency waves and with continuity toward greater diversity and complexity. To say that man's patterns of relating are rhythmical means that they are characterized by a complex of wave forms and resonances, the qualities of which are timing and flowing.[35] The timing and flowing qualities describe a rhythm. Timing refers to the cadence evident in a recurrent beat. It is sometimes fast, sometimes slow, but ever evolving universally toward shorter, higher-frequency waves, thus faster rhythms,[36] like a rubber ball dropped on a hard surface that returns a shorter distance on each successive rebound and does so at a perceptibly faster speed each time. Flowing refers to the metrical continuity evident as the changing beats become more diverse and more complex, like waves of the sea, moving onward with the alternating rise and fall, somewhat the same yet becoming different with each movement of wave with wave and more complex with each movement of wave with sea. Timing and flowing are evident in the rhythmical patterns of Man-Living-Health. For example, as person-to-person interchange becomes more frequent between two individuals who care about each other, it becomes more intense (higher-frequency waves) and thus the rhythm becomes faster each time the couple meets. Each is more diverse and more complex than before in that each has evolved through other experiences since their last meeting. Rhythmic patterns of relating are com-

[35] George B. Leonard, *The Silent Pulse* (New York: E. P. Dutton, 1978), p. xii.

[36] Martha E. Rogers, "Nursing: A Science of Unitary Man," in *Conceptual Models for Nursing Practice*, eds. Joan P. Riehl and Callista Roy (New York: Appleton-Century-Crofts, 1980), p. 331.

plementary and are lived all at once in situation. This means that apparent opposite rhythmic patterns are present simultaneously. For example, a person choosing a commitment to an ideal simultaneously gives up another possible commitment. The specific concepts of this principle are rhythms of Man-Living-Health, revealing-concealing, enabling-limiting, and connecting-separating. These are described next.

Revealing-Concealing

Revealing-concealing, the first concept, is a recognizable rhythmic pattern of Man-Living-Health. It is the simultaneous disclosing of some aspects of self and hiding of others. Fundamental to this rhythm, for Buber, is the idea of being and seeming, the duality of the interhuman. Being is the way a man knows self; seeming is the way man portrays self to others.[37] This is foundational for Buber in that he believes man chooses to reveal and conceal all at once in interrelationships with others. This revealing-concealing pattern uncovers man as more than and different from that which is seen by others. There is always more to a person than what the other experiences in the immediate situation. There is always that which is simultaneously concealed. Marcel agrees with Buber when he discusses presence.[38] He says there is always mystery present, that which cannot be readily ascertained about a person, that which is simultaneously hidden. Jourard concurs with Buber and Marcel when he discusses disclosing and not disclosing as the way man relates to man.[39] He states that self-disclosure involves courage and that in the process

[37] Martin Buber, *The Knowledge of Man*, ed. Maurice Friedman (New York: Harper & Row, 1965), p. 75.

[38] Gabriel Marcel, *Mystery of Being: Reflection and Mystery*, vol. I (South Bend, Indiana: Gateway Editions, 1978), pp. 207–212.

[39] Sidney M. Jourard, *Transparent Self* (New York: Van Nostrand Reinhold, 1964), p. 3.

of becoming known to another one gains knowledge of self.[40] The rhythm of disclosing-not disclosing for Jourard is involved with choosing and being authentic and is a reflection of health.[41] The rhythmic pattern of revealing-concealing then flows in cadence between man and man as a recognizable feature of Man-Living-Health.

Enabling-Limiting

Enabling-limiting is another rhythmical pattern of Man-Living-Health. It shows that man in situation is simultaneously enabled and limited. Enabling-limiting is evident as man chooses to be certain ways in situation. In this choosing, man enables self to move in one direction and limits movement in another. Sartre states that man is fundamentally free and chooses to be a certain way in situation.[42] In fact, man must continuously make choices. Every event in the world is man's opportunity to choose.[43] Merleau-Ponty agrees with Sartre, and he states that man is "open to an infinite number of possibilities . . . ."[44] Man cannot be all possibilities at once, and, in choosing, one is both enabled and limited. There is a recognizable flow and cadence to the enabling-limiting in Man-Living-Health.

Connecting-Separating

Connecting-separating, the third concept of cocreating rhythmical patterns of relating, can be recognized as

[40] Ibid., p. 11.

[41] Ibid., p. 24.

[42] Jean-Paul Sartre, *Being and Nothingness* (New York: Washington Square Press, 1966), p. 574.

[43] Ibid., p. 711.

[44] Maurice Merleau-Ponty, *Phenomenology of Perception* (New York: Humanities Press, 1974), p. 453.

man is connecting with one phenomenon and simultaneously separating from others. Connecting-separating is discussed by a number of theorists who generally give this rhythmic pattern similar meaning but name it differently. Unifying and separating is a happening, according to Kempler, who says that each separating leads to a higher order of union and the process of separating and unifying is the "main thrust of human development."[45]

Two or more people come together in an intersubjective relationship; that is, they are truly present to each other, simultaneously unifying and separating as their togetherness evolves. While these individuals are participating with each other, they all at once are separating from others.

In separating from one phenomenon and dwelling with another, a person integrates thought, becomes more complex, and seeks new unions. Buber concurs with Kempler in a general sense. Buber's view is that the two-fold principle of human life is distancing and relating. He believes that one can enter into a relationship only with that which one has set at a distance.[46] When relating with one phenomenon, others are set at a distance. van Kaam, et al. say "man is a rhythm of communion and aloneness. . . ."[47] Both aspects of the rhythm are a source of human unfolding. Participation or communion is being involved with the activity at hand while simultaneously not being involved with other activities. Moving away from the activity at hand is simultaneously moving toward another activity. This rhythmic pattern confirms man as uniquely unifying and separating all at once. In everyday living with people and with environment, man is simultaneously

[45] Walter Kempler, *Principles of Gestalt Family Therapy* (Oslo, Norway, A. S. Nordales, Trykkert, 1974), p. 65.

[46] Buber, *Knowledge of Man*, p. 80.

[47] Adrian van Kaam, Bert van Croonenburg, and Susan Muto, *The Participant Self*, vol. II (Pittsburgh: Duquesne University Press), p. 30.

close to some phenomena and distant from others. This is a continuous cadent process and a feature of Man-Living-Health.

The rhythmic patterns of relating, revealing-concealing, enabling-limiting, and connecting-separating just described are seen in everyday life experiences as identifiable characteristics of Man-Living-Health. For example, a family—Mr. and Mrs. Baker, 15-year-old Jim, and 10-year-old Sharon—has chosen to jog together twice a week. This activity is a way of *connecting* the family as a unit while *separating* the family from other persons and phenomena. Within the family method of jogging, such as who runs next to whom, there can also be seen a *connection* of two or more family members while simultaneously *separating* them from others. The family running session *enables* and *limits* all at once in that it *enables* family togetherness while *limiting* other activities for its members, perhaps golf, swimming, or football. The choosing of one activity for now *limits* participating in another. Jogging together as a family *reveals* a value for jogging and being together but simultaneously *conceals* the value for other activities as well as the meaning of jogging and being together for each family member. Cocreating rhythmical patterns of relating is exemplified in the Baker family's jogging together, and this is a reflection of Man-Living-Health.

PRINCIPLE 3: COTRANSCENDING WITH THE POSSIBLES IS POWERING UNIQUE WAYS OF ORIGINATING IN THE PROCESS OF TRANSFORMING

This principle means that Man-Living-Health is powering original transformation through coconstituting with others. Man aspires toward that which is not-yet and reaches beyond toward the future.[48] This reaching beyond does not mean beyond experience; it means living several modes of experience all at once.[49] Man exists with others and in this interrelationship continues to cocreate self and chooses to make possibles actuals. The actuals are the contextual situations that man has cocreated. The possibles arise from the context of the situations as opportunities from which alternatives are chosen. New actuals create other possibles, and, in this way, man continuously chooses ways of being while cotranscending with the possibles. Human existence is such that man is coconstituting the situation and simultaneously cotranscending it. Through multidimensional experiences, man is aware of other possibles. This is related to man's freedom in situation. "By transcending the given situation . . . man frees himself within certain limits from the situation. This opens up alternatives; the dimension of actuality is left behind and the realm of potentiality is entered, creating the possibility of choice and the necessity of decision. . . ."[50] Man's orientation toward the possible is revealed in powering and cocreating that which is beyond self in indefinite space and time.[51]

Cotranscending, then, is the way man with environment reaches beyond and propels into the future.[52] Cotranscending with the possibles is powering originating toward transforming. The concepts of cotranscending with the possibles are powering, originating, and transforming. These will be discussed separately.

[48] Merleau-Ponty, *Phenomenology of Perception*, p. 421.

[49] Marcel, *Mystery of Being*, vol I, pp. 39-56.

[50] Walter A. Weisskopf, "Existence and Values," in *New Knowledge in Human Values*, ed. A. H. Maslow (Chicago: Henry Regnery Company, 1959), p. 109.

[51] Maurice Merleau-Ponty, *The Structure of Behavior* (Boston: Beacon Press, 1963), pp. 175-176.

[52] Viktor E. Frankl, *The Will to Meaning* (New York: New American Library, 1959), p. 55.

Powering

Powering is the first concept of cotranscending with the possibles. "It originates when we turn towards the future which happens in different ways; in dreams of future happiness, in the play of imagination with possibilities, in hesitations, and in fear. . . ."[53] Since man's orientation is toward the future, powering is fundamental to being.[54] It is the force of human existence and underpins the courage to be.[55] That man exists means man is powering. One cannot not power. Powering is a process of man-environment energy interchange, recognized in the continuous affirming of self in light of the possibility of non-being. Being is continuously confronted with non-being. Non-being shows itself in everyday life as man risks losing self in man-other interrelationships. The risk of losing self here refers not only to dying but to the risk of losing one's self through being rejected, threatened, or not recognized in a manner consistent with expectations. Powering is a continuous rhythmical process incarnating one's intentions and actions in moving toward possibilities.[56] Pushing-resisting is the rhythm of powering that occurs all at once "in every moment of life in all relations of all beings . . . between man and nature, between man and man, between individuals and groups, between groups and groups."[57]

Powering patterns unfold in man-other interrelationships and show themselves through languaging. Every encounter is a struggle of powering with powering. The struggle is languaged through gesture, gaze, touch, ver-

[53] Dilthey, *Pattern and Meaning in History*, p. 109.

[54] Paul Tillich, *Love, Power and Justice* (New York: Oxford University Press, 1954), p. 37.

[55] Paul Tillich, *The Courage to Be* (New Haven: Yale University Press, 1952), p. 3.

[56] Dilthey, *Pattern and Meaning in History*, p. 110.

[57] Tillich, *Love, Power and Justice*, p. 42.

balization, intonation, and what one represents person-
ally and socially.[58] Powering is evidenced in being present with the world. How one lives powering is reflected
in one's patterns of relating with the world through the
rhythm of pushing-resisting. Pushing-resisting is present
in every human encounter, creating tension and sometimes conflict. Possibles unfold through the tension and
conflict that create the alternatives from which one
can choose in reaching beyond. Tension is the struggling
between pushing and resisting while contending with
others, issues, ideas, desires, and hopes all at once in
the process of striving to reach new possibles. In the
struggling an individual emerges in cotranscending
toward what is not-yet.

Conflict surfaces in situation when the tension between pushing and resisting is changed, opening the way
for opposition between worldviews relative to issues.
Conflict is the opposition. It offers opportunities for
individuals to examine the worldviews of others in
situation and make choices with others to move beyond
to new possibles. Powering is a process in all change
and transformation from what one is to what one is not-
yet. For example, the Cook family, a husband and
wife with one child, have a pattern of relating in which
Mrs. Cook makes decisions and Mr. Cook generally
agrees. They discover, after living the tension of *pushing-
resisting*, that their worldviews differ about their child's
discipline relative to scholastic performance. Mrs. Cook
believes strongly in using incentives such as extra
money and new material acquisitions to encourage
better scholastic performance, and this becomes the
course of action with the child and Mr. Cook quietly
agrees. The Cook family lives the *pushing-resisting*
tension pattern for a period of time. Mrs. Cook continually encourages the child to perform better through
offering material goods. This is pushing emphasizing

[58] Ibid., p. 87.

her worldview while at the same time it is a *resisting* of her husband's view. Mr. Cook's silence is *pushing* in that it pushes Mrs. Cook to continue the discipline strategy. He is simultaneously *resisting* the opportunity to initiate a new struggle and change the discipline strategy. These individual powering patterns of Mr. and Mrs. Cook with their child unfold in the day-to-day living of this decision. Mr. Cook, who quietly agreed to the arrangement, remains silent while Mrs. Cook struggles in conversation with the child relative to the rewards for scholastic performance. Mrs. Cook, whose idea it was to discipline in this way, experiences frustration that she languages with gestures, intonations, and facial expressions. Mr. Cook remains silent, and the struggle of powering with powering is apparent. The struggling continues, and the Cook family emerges as the child's scholastic performance becomes an issue for the parents. Mr. Cook decides to participate no longer in the original decision by remaining silent. The *pushing-resisting* rhythm is changed and conflict surfaces. The parents confront their worldviews as different and new alternatives, such as restrict-the child, combining restricting and incentives, as well as others, arise. The new possibles bring to the surface new ways of viewing the situation, and powering struggles with powering as each parent affirms self over non-being, that is, the threat of not having his or her own values lived in the family. Through this struggle, the family cotranscends toward what is not-yet. In this way powering is an essence of cotranscending with the possibles and is foundational to transforming. It is an everyday occurrence and a recognizable feature of Man-Living-Health.

Originating

Originating is the second concept chosen to illuminate cotranscending with the possibles. Originating is a continuing process of negentropically unfolding while emerging in mutual energy interchange with the environment. It is choosing a particular way of self-emergence through inventing unique ways of living. Powering ways of originating is man distinguishing self from others.[59] To distinguish oneself is to choose a unique way of living the paradoxical unity of conformity-nonconformity and certainty-uncertainty all at once. The paradoxical unity of conformity-nonconformity surfaces in human encounters, as individuals seek to be like others yet, simultaneously, not to be like others. Seeking to be like others is to focus on the commonalities in self and others while moving toward making oneself comfortable and attempting to share responsibility.[60] Seeking to be different is to focus on that which is distinct in self. It is a way of confirming autonomy and uniqueness. The paradox of living certainty-uncertainty surfaces in human encounter as individuals make concrete or clear their choices in situation yet, simultaneously, live the ambiguity of the unknown outcomes. In human encounters individuals continuously are called on by others to be more conforming and less unique while moving toward that which is more certain than uncertain; when each defines certainty and conformity in the same way, then all strive for commonness. There may be more comfort in sameness and more safety in certainty. The *kind* of certainty-uncertainty and conformity-nonconformity, rather than the *degree*, is related to one's patterns of originating. One does not have *more* or *less* certainty or conformity but rather certainty and conformity in relation to the context of the situation. Originating then springs from transcending

[59] Friedrich Nietzsche, *The Will to Power*, ed. W. Kaufmann (New York: Vintage Books, 1968), p. 412.

[60] Adrian van Kaam, Bert van Croonenburg, and Susan Muto, *The Emergent Self* (Wilkes-Barre, Pennsylvania: Dimension Books, 1968), p. 45.

these paradoxes in day-to-day human encounters. To transcend the paradoxes one images new possibles, thus opening up "vast opportunities for inventing novel connections and seeing unusual analogies"[61] for originating transformation. With a particular decision, one seeks a vision of the whole structure, a completed picture of what living the decision would mean. The vision of the whole structure moves one to be more comfortable while affirming self as unique, thus living the paradoxical unity of conformity-nonconformity. The idea of the whole structure also moves one to make clear the choices while envisioning the anticipated outcomes, yet with the ambiguity of not knowing the *actual* outcomes in living the paradox of certainty-uncertainty. This process of originating is coconstituted in man-other interrelationships. One's patterns of originating emerge in this interrelationship and are languaged through one's ways of relating. Conformity-nonconformity and certainty-uncertainty are patterns of originating in situation.

For example, The Daly family, Mr. and Mrs. Daly and their son, Mike, are confronted with the decision of choosing a university for Mike. In the human encounter of decision making relative to this issue, the family patterns of originating surface. The family has many options, since Mike is an acceptable candidate for many universities. From the many options the family co-creates the image, the whole structure of Mike attending an Ivy League school. This moves the Daly family to be comfortable in seeking some common ground with Ivy League families while affirming itself as a unique and autonomous family, living *conformity-nonconformity* all at once. Mike would be the only member of his graduating class and of his generational family to attend an Ivy League school. The whole structure with the visioned outcomes—Mike would perform well

---

[61] Bruteau, *The Psychic Grid*, p. 219.

enough to remain in school; investments would be lucrative enough to finance his education; and the family's social class would be enhanced—moves the family to apply for Mike's admission, knowing the ambiguity relative to the various possible outcomes. This is living the paradox of *certainty-uncertainty*. Through this process of originating, the family becomes more complex as it invents new ways of living the patterns of conformity-nonconformity and certainty-uncertainty. In this way, originating relates to cotranscending with the possibles and is a recognizable feature of Man-Living-Health.

Transforming

The third concept of cotranscending with the possibles is transforming. Transforming is the changing of change, coconstituting anew in a deliberate way. In the man-environment interrelationship, change is an ongoing process; that is, man coparticipates with environment in the simultaneous unfolding called change.

This unfolding reveals itself in everyday life as man continually participates with the environment in co-creating becoming. Innovative discoveries and shifts in worldview are coconstituted through the simultaneous interchange between person and world. The person is open to the discovery, and the phenomenon is open to be discovered. The opportunity for discovery then emerges in the context of the person-world interrelationship. This idea is supported by van den Berg in his theory of changes. van den Berg believes that discoveries surfacing at a given moment are directly related to both the ongoing changes in human existence and the simultaneous changes in the world over time.[62]

[62] J. H. van den Berg, "Phenomenology and Metabletics," *Humanitas*, 7 (3), 1971, p. 285.

He believes in a person-world "changeable together-ness" which in itself surfaces unique possibilities for discovery.[63]

These unique possibilities unfold in the person-world interrelationship through a rhythmical process of struggling to integrate the unfamiliar with the familiar. In the process of transforming, a person increases in complexity through integrating new discoveries and continuously becoming the not-yet. Threads of consistency are apparent in this process of integrating, confirming the simultaneous presence of who one is, was, and will become. This simultaneous presence is the unity of cocreated relationships that form a person's patterns of relating.[64] The individual is recognized through these patterns that incarnate chosen values in a coherent connectedness of the familiar-unfamiliar. Dilthey reflects on this when he says, "The person who seeks the connecting threads in the history of his life has already, from different points of view, created a coherence in that life . . . by experiencing values and realizing purposes. . . ."[65] In the process of transforming, then, a person experiences struggling and leaping beyond in continuous movement toward greater complexity.

The ongoing process of change has been described by Watzlawick et al., in a two-level framework, as first-order and second-order change. First-order change occurs within the system itself without changing the structure of that system. Types of first-order change are change by exception, increment, and pendulum shift.[66] Second-order change is a change in the structure

[63] Ibid., p. 288.

[64] Dilthey, *Pattern and Meaning in History*, p. 103.

[65] Ibid., p. 86.

[66] Ferguson, *The Aquarian Conspiracy*, p. 71.

of the system itself.[67] It is a whole pattern change, a transforming of the nature of the system.

Consistent with Watzlawick's definition of second-order change is Ferguson's definition of transforming as the "fourth dimension of change: the new perspective, the insight that allows the information to come together in a new form or structure."[68] It is a deliberate shift in one's way of viewing the familiar.[69] Man by nature is open to transforming.[70] The possibilities of transforming or shifting one's views emerge in the process of discovering self in situation. Perspectives of self emerge in human encounters as individuals view themselves as well as view themselves being viewed by others. One's view of the other's view of self is a metaperspective.[71] One's view of the other's view of the view is a meta metaperspective.[72] These various perspectives unfold the discovering of self and cocreate the possibilities of transforming. As one experiences these perspectives in the gaze, dialogue, and touch of others, the realization of what one envisions he is not, for self and others, simultaneously emerges with what one envisions one is and can become. Discovering perspectives of self that were previously present only in prereflective awareness opens a person to a different way of viewing the familiar, the creating of a different meaning of a situation. Creating a different meaning is changing the conceptual viewpoint relative to a situation, that is, placing it in another light that

---

[67] Paul Watzlawick, John Weakland, and Richard Fisch, *Change: Principles of Problem Formation and Problem Resolution* (New York: W. W. Norton, 1974), p. 10.

[68] Ferguson, *The Aquarian Conspiracy*, p. 72.

[69] Watzlawick, Weakland, and Fisch, *Change*, p. 9.

[70] Ferguson, *The Aquarian Conspiracy*, p. 29.

[71] R. D. Laing, H. Phillipson, and A. R. Lee, *Interpersonal Perception: A Theory and a Method of Research* (New York: Harper & Row, 1966), pp. 5-6.

[72] Ibid.

fits the facts of the same situation, thereby changing its entire meaning.[73] The meaning changes as the different perspectives shed new light on the situation. New light is shed, as a burst of insight illuminates the situation from a different vantage point.[74] This shift to a different vantage point is a shift in one's changing worldview, a changing of change. This changing of change is transforming, deliberately choosing a new worldview and, in so doing, a new way of being. Man's continuous transforming is self-initiated and creative.

Once a person has chosen the experience of a shift to new insight, he cannot return to viewing self in a situation in the old way but can only move toward other possibles. For example, the Evans family—consisting of Mr. and Mrs. Evans and three teenage children, Barry, Patty, and Lucy—exemplifies transforming as it relates to Man-Living-Health. Mr. Evans consults with the family but is generally responsible for major family decisions. This is the Evans family pattern of decision making. Mrs. Evans's mother, Mrs. Olds, is 76 and self-sufficient. Recently she has been complaining of a lack of energy. After a complete medical examination, the physician made no specific diagnosis for the "draggy feeling with no pep" that Mrs. Olds expressed frequently. The family talked with Mrs. Olds about her apparent lack of enthusiasm for life, lack of desire to cook for herself and maintain a residence, and her apparent search for a reason to live. The Evans family discussed the possibilities for Mrs. Olds, one of which was to invite her to live with them. All the members of the Evans family agreed that Mrs. Olds wanted to be needed and to have a purpose in life. The option to have Mrs. Olds move in with the Evans family was viewed by Mr. Evans, Barry, and Lucy as an intrusion on their life-style. Barry and Lucy

[73] Watzlawick, Weakland, and Fisch, *Change*, p. 95.
[74] Ferguson, *The Aquarian Conspiracy*, p. 68.

said that it would interfere with parties and other activities in the home. Mr. Evans thought that Mrs. Evans would "tie herself down" if her mother moved into the family home. Mrs. Evans and Patty talked with Mr. Evans, Barry, and Lucy at length about their way of being with the situation. Mrs. Olds had often participated in the Evans family's life in earlier years, especially when the children were young and Mrs. Olds was needed for help. The family members' perspectives of each other surfaced in the discussion and prompted each member to contemplate how he or she was viewed by others in this group, and the decision about Mrs. Olds moving into the Evans home became an important issue for the family. Mr. Evans began seriously to consider his wife's way of looking at him, prompted primarily by the comment that "Mom was 'good old Mom' when we needed her so that I could participate in your business endeavors—I just can't believe you are resisting helping my mother now—I've never known you this way." Mr. Evans saw himself being seen differently by Mrs. Evans. He then saw himself differently. He spoke with the children about the issue. Barry and Lucy said, "Hold your ground, Dad. Grandma's great, but to live with us is another story." The usually quiet Patty winced when she said, "Dad, we have to help Grandma." Mr. Evans saw what Mrs. Evans and the children said he was not and also possibilities of who he could become. He began to consider the perspectives of himself that surfaced in this situation that had not surfaced before. Mr. Evans was open to creating a different meaning in this situation. He had further discussions with Mrs. Evans, and one afternoon he said to a close friend who joined the family for lunch, "We're talking about having my mother-in-law live with us. I don't know about such a move." The friend immediately said, "Oh, you mean Mrs. Olds will be moving in to help manage the household so you and your wife can be free to travel and expand your business. What a help she'll be with your kids. You're lucky," Mr. Evans said, "Well, I hadn't thought about it quite that way." Mr. Evans's view of the friend's view of the situation created a different meaning for him. The other family members also began to consider the situation in a new light, one that focused attention on the asset Mrs. Olds could be to the family. After much discussion on the new meaning, Mrs. Olds was invited to move into the Evans's to participate in managing the household. In the excitement of moving in with the Evans family, Mrs. Olds's energy patterns changed. She had a new spark and lightness. She said she was delighted with the opportunity to help manage the Evans household.

The transforming emerged in the human encounters of the Evans family members with a friend as their various perspectives surfaced and cocreated the possibility for a new meaning in this situation. The family was open to a new view of the situation, and the situation was open to be viewed in a new way. The new meaning shifted a worldview, changing the family's way of being with Mrs. Olds's moving into the Evans's family home. Transforming, a concept of cotranscending with the possibles, is a recognizable feature of Man-Living-Health.

The three principles just discussed, with their essential concepts, describe Man-Living-Health. Man-Living-Health is structuring meaning multidimensionally in cocreating rhythmical patterns of relating while cotranscending with the possibles. Man-Living-Health, man becoming, is the day-to-day creating of reality through the languaging of valuing and imaging. Languaging reflects the rhythms of revealing-concealing, enabling-limiting, and connecting-separating as people live powering as a way of originating transforming.

Man participates in creating health by choosing the imaged values in multidimensional experiences that become man's way of relating with the world. Man's way of relating is through the rhythmical patterns of revealing-concealing, enabling-limiting, and connecting-separating. These rhythms are lived as man comes to know, prize values, and language symbols in the struggle with paradoxes toward transformation of self. This is Man-Living-Health.

The principles and concepts of Man-Living-Health give rise to theoretical structures. A theoretical structure is a statement interrelating concepts in a way that can be verified. Some emergent theoretical structures of Man-Living-Health are

- *Theoretical Structure 1*: Powering is a way of revealing and concealing imaging.
- *Theoretical Structure 2*: Originating is a manifestation of enabling and limiting valuing.
- *Theoretical Structure 3*: Transforming unfolds in the languaging of connecting and separating.

Schema 6 shows the emergence of the theoretical structures. Other structures may be generated from this design. Schema 7 depicts the evolution of the theory of Man-Living-Health.

SUMMARY

Man-Living-Health is a theory of nursing grounded in the human sciences. It is based on assumptions that were synthesized from principles, tenets, and concepts from the works of Martha E. Rogers and several existential-phenomenologists. The three principles, nine concepts, and three theoretical structures of Man-Living-Health follow.

SCHEMA 6. RELATIONSHIP OF PRINCIPLES, CONCEPTS, AND THEORETICAL STRUCTURES OF MAN-LIVING-HEALTH

Principle 1: Structuring meaning multidimensionally is cocreating reality through the languaging of valuing and imaging.

Principle 2: Cocreating rhythmical patterns of relating is living the paradoxical unity of revealing-concealing and enabling-limiting while connecting-separating.

Principle 3: Cotranscending with the possibles is powering unique ways of originating in the process of transforming.

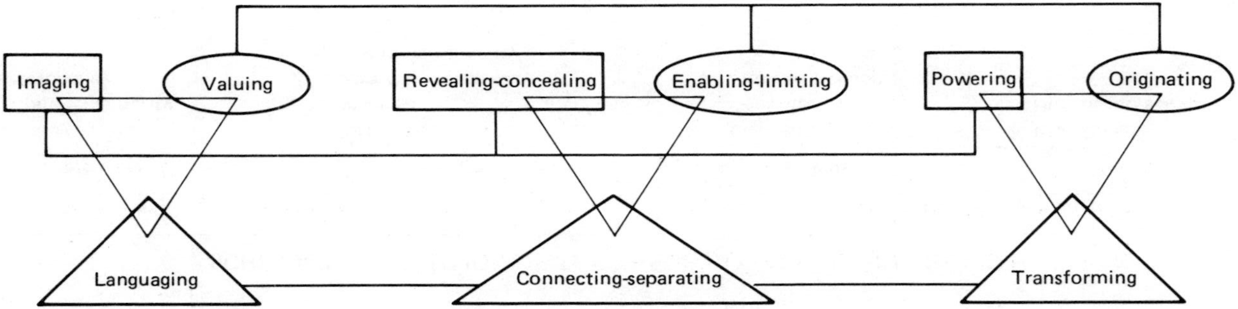

Relationship of the concepts in the *squares:* *Powering* is a way of *revealing and concealing imaging.*
Relationship of the concepts in the *ovals:* *Originating* is a manifestation of *enabling and limiting valuing.*
Relationship of the concepts in the *triangles:* *Transforming* unfolds in the *languaging of connecting and separating.*

69

SCHEMA 7. EVOLUTION OF THE THEORY OF MAN-LIVING-HEALTH

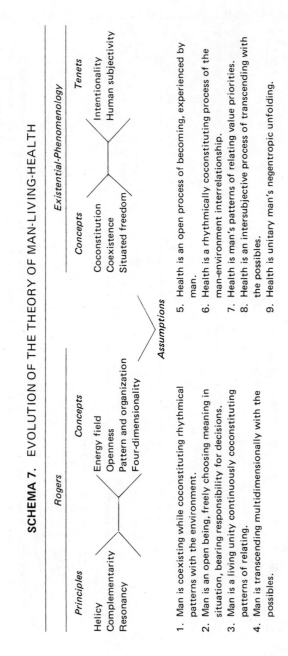

Rogers

Principles

Helicy
Complementarity
Resonancy

Concepts

Energy field
Openness
Pattern and organization
Four-dimensionality

Existential-Phenomenology

Concepts

Coconstitution
Coexistence
Situated freedom

Tenets

Intentionality
Human subjectivity

Assumptions

1. Man is coexisting while coconstituting rhythmical patterns with the environment.
2. Man is an open being, freely choosing meaning in situation, bearing responsibility for decisions.
3. Man is a living unity continuously coconstituting patterns of relating.
4. Man is transcending multidimensionally with the possibles.
5. Health is an open process of becoming, experienced by man.
6. Health is a rhythmically coconstituting process of the man-environment interrelationship.
7. Health is man's patterns of relating value priorities.
8. Health is an intersubjective process of transcending with the possibles.
9. Health is unitary man's negentropic unfolding.

Man-Living-Health

	Structuring meaning multidimensionally	Cocreating rhythmical patterns of relating	Cotranscending with the possibles
Principles			
Concepts	Imaging Valuing Languaging	Revealing-concealing Enabling-limiting Connecting-separating	Powering Originating Transforming
Theoretical Structures	*Powering* is a way of *revealing and concealing imaging.* *Originating* is a manifestation of *enabling and limiting valuing.* *Transforming* unfolds in the *languaging of connecting and separating.*		

- *Principle 1*: Structuring meaning multidimensionally
    Concepts:
        Imaging
        Valuing
        Languaging
- *Principle 2*: Cocreating rhythmical patterns of relating
    Concepts:
        Revealing-concealing
        Enabling-limiting
        Connecting-separating
- *Principle 3*: Cotranscending with the possibles
    Concepts:
        Powering
        Originating
        Transforming

Some theoretical structures emerging from the inter-relationship of these principles and concepts are

- *Theoretical Structure 1*: Powering is a way of revealing and concealing imaging.
- *Theoretical Structure 2*: Originating is a manifestation of enabling and limiting valuing.
- *Theoretical Structure 3*: Transforming unfolds in the languaging of connecting and separating.

Schema 8 depicts the theory of Man-Living-Health.

SCHEMA 8. THE THEORY OF MAN-LIVING-HEALTH

Assumptions

1. Man is coexisting while coconstituting rhythmical patterns with the environment.
2. Man is an open being, freely choosing meaning in situation, bearing responsibility for decisions.
3. Man is a living unity continuously coconstituting patterns of relating.
4. Man is transcending multidimensionally with the possibles.
5. Health is an open process of becoming, experienced by man.
6. Health is a rhythmically coconstituting process of the man-environment interrelationship.
7. Health is man's patterns of relating value priorities.
8. Health is an intersubjective process of transcending with the possibles.
9. Health is unitary man's negentropic unfolding.

Man-Living-Health

	Principles	
Principles	Structuring meaning multidimensionally	Cocreating rhythmical patterns of relating	Cotranscending with the possibles
Concepts	Imaging	Revealing-concealing	Powering
	Valuing	Enabling-limiting	Originating
	Languaging	Connecting-separating	Transforming

Theoretical Structures

Powering is a way of revealing and concealing *imaging.*
Originating is a manifestation of enabling and limiting *valuing.*
Transforming unfolds in the *languaging of connecting and separating.*

CHAPTER V

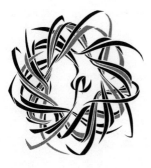

Empirical Aspects of Man-Living-Health: A Theory of Nursing

■

THEORY, RESEARCH, PRACTICE, AND EDUCATION

The interrelationship among theory, research, practice, and education is foundational to the evolution of nursing as a science and an art. Theory creatively invented from a conceptual system is verified through scholarly research. The findings of research enhance the theory and the conceptual system, expanding the body of nursing knowledge. The body of nursing knowledge is the theoretical base that guides nursing practice. As the changing man-environment interrelationship creates new discoveries in nursing practice, implications for research are uncovered that, when pursued, enhance nursing's knowledge base. The body of nursing knowledge is reflected in the content of the nursing curricula in baccalaureate, master's, and doctoral programs. The doctoral curriculum, particularly, focuses on nursing research, providing educational guidance for those preparing to be leaders in enhancing the knowledge base of nursing. The interrelationship among theory, research, practice, and education is a synergistic process in the evolution of nursing as a science and art rooted in its own body of knowledge. The specific empirical implications of *Man-Living-Health: A Theory of Nursing* presented in Chapter IV are discussed next.

IMPLICATIONS FOR RESEARCH

Man-Living-Health: A Theory of Nursing, described in Chapter IV, invites empirical verification. The theory, rooted in the human sciences, describes health as man's coparticipation in becoming. It is expected that this theory will be verified through descriptive methodologies, an example of which is the phenomenological method. The phenomenological method is "defined as the study of phenomena . . . in the way these phenomena appear."[1] This methodology is a rigorous inductive process of uncovering a structure of meaning of lived experiences. A detailed description of the method is outlined by Spiegelberg in *The Phenomenological Movement.*[2] The structures of meaning of lived experiences in themselves will enhance this theory of nursing in that, from the perspective of this theory, all lived experiences are related to Man-Living-Health. It is expected that structures of meaning of lived experiences will be developed through the descriptive methodologies and will enhance the knowledge base of Man-Living-Health. This theory of nursing, then, grounded in the human sciences, will be enhanced by verification through descriptive methodologies.

Examples of some phenomena that might be studied in relation to this theory are listed next in relation to the theoretical structures.

THEORETICAL STRUCTURE 1 :
POWERING IS A WAY OF REVEALING
AND CONCEALING IMAGING

Some lived experiences that might be studied in relation to this theoretical structure are "struggling with uncovering hidden meanings in a dialogue" and "struggling in creating possibilities for self-disclosure." Descriptions

[1] J. H. van den Berg, "Phenomenology and Metabletics," *Humanitas* 7 (3), 1971, p. 283.

[2] Herbert Speigelberg, *The Phenomenological Movement,* vols. I and II (The Hague, Netherlands: Martinus Nijhoff, 1976).

that subjects might be asked to share relative to these lived experiences follow.

Lived Experience	*Description*
Struggling with uncovering the hidden meaning in a dialogue	Describe a situation in which you experienced yourself struggling to clarify the ambiguous messages in a conversation.
Struggling in cocreating possibilities for self-disclosure	Describe a situation in which you experienced yourself being listened to.

THEORETICAL STRUCTURE 2: ORIGINATING IS A MANIFESTATION OF ENABLING AND LIMITING VALUING

Some lived experiences that might be studied in relation to this theoretical structure are "being enabled and limited by a choice" and "being different from others." Descriptions that subjects might be asked to share relative to these lived experiences follow.

Lived Experience	*Description*
Being enabled and limited by a choice	Describe a situation in which you experienced yourself making an important decision.
Being different from others	Describe a situation in which you experienced yourself taking an unpopular stand on an issue.

THEORETICAL STRUCTURE 3:
TRANSFORMING UNFOLDS IN THE
LANGUAGING OF CONNECTING
AND SEPARATING

Some lived experiences that might be studied in relation
to this theoretical structure are "planning for the
future" and "shifting points of view." Descriptions
that subjects might be asked to share relative to these
lived experiences follow.

Lived Experience	*Description*
Planning for the future	Describe a situation in which you experienced yourself anticipating an upcoming event.
Shifting points of view	Describe a situation in which you experienced yourself having new insight into a familiar issue.

   The structures of meaning that are uncovered in the
phenomenological study of these and other lived experiences will enhance the theory of Man-Living-Health.
Research studies to verify the theory of nursing posited
in this book are already being developed relative to the
preceding phenomena. Examples of these studies are
the lived experiences of "feeling rested," "living with
ambiguity," and "discovering."

IMPLICATIONS FOR PRACTICE

Man-Living-Health: A Theory of Nursing, described in
Chapter IV, invites pragmatic verification in the world
of nursing practice. The practice of nursing involves

both the science and the art. It is the utilization of nursing's abstract body of knowledge in service to people. From the perspective of the theory articulated in this book, nursing's responsibility is to society. The responsibility to society relative to nursing practice is guiding the choosing of possibilities in the changing health process. This guiding is through the intersubjective participation with persons and their families. Family is defined as the others with whom one is closely connected. Nursing practice is innovative and creative, unencumbered by prescriptive rules. The principles of the theory of Man-Living-Health provide a broad base of abstract nursing knowledge that guides nursing practice. The principle of structuring meaning multidimensionally posits that Man-Living-Health in relation to others structures reality. Man's reality is the languaging of imaged values chosen from options in multidimensional experiences.

The meaning man assigns to situations reveals and conceals imaged hopes and desires. Living health is languaging all at once the chosen explicit reality and the mystery of that which lies hidden in tacit knowing. Health is each person's unique experience of valuing. One's perspective of health, then, can be known only through a personal description even though it is co-created through interrelationships with others. The principle of structuring meaning multidimensionally guides nursing practice to focus on illuminating unique ways in which generational and contemporary family interrelationships cocreate lived values. This principle further guides practice to focus on mobilizing family energies for structuring and languaging different meanings in light of family health possibilities.

The principle of cocreating rhythmical patterns of relating specifies the open energy interchange between man and environment as rhythmical patterns of revealing-concealing, enabling-limiting, and connecting-separating. These patterns are lived all at once as characteristic of Man-Living-Health. Man's patterns of relating reflect in languaging the value priorities of the changing health process. The principle of cocreating rhythmical patterns of relating guides nursing practice to focus on illuminating the family patterns of interrelating in light of the changing value priorities in the family's living of health. Family awareness of patterns of relating enhances opportunities for the changing of health patterns.

The principle of cotranscending with the possibles specifies that man is continuously changing through a process of struggling, leaping ahead, and struggling anew. This process is reflective of man's living the paradoxical unity of conformity, certainty, familiarity, and pushing all at once. Man-Living-Health is the transforming of values through reaching beyond to other possibilities. This principle, cotranscending with the possibles, guides nursing practice to focus on mobilizing family energies in reflectively choosing shifts in viewpoints relative to the possibilities available in the changing health process.

The principles of Man-Living-Health, then, guide nursing practice in a unique way. Paramount in this theory is man's participation in and perspective of health as it is cocreated through interrelationships with others. Nursing practice is directed toward illuminating and mobilizing family interrelationships in light of the meaning assigned to health and its possibilities as languaged in the cocreated patterns of relating. Nursing practice is continuously changing as the abstract body of nursing knowledge is expanded through scholarly research.

An example of a family situation follows with discussion related to the theory of Man-Living-Health. The description of the family situation, the decision-making pattern, and the family's contextual situation emerged from meetings between the family and nurse. The nurse participated with the family through illuminating patterns and mobilizing energies toward the changing health perspectives evident as the situation unfolded.

Family Situation

Mr. and Mrs. Taylor have two children: Randy, age 18, and Jamie, age 14.

PROFILE OF MR. TAYLOR

From His Perspective

- Ultra conservative and frugal
- Has a traditional belief system, for example:
  - Women are fragile, weak, and need a man's protection.
  - Children must honor and obey their parents.
- Works hard as a comptroller for a large corporation
- Breadwinner

From Randy's Perspective

- Strict but fair
- Sometimes difficult to talk with
- Would like to be like him

*From Mrs. Taylor's
Perspective*

- Her best friend
- Strong, provides well
  for the family
- Strict with the
  children
- Could be more
  flexible
- Handsome
- Enjoys being with
  friends

From Jamie's Perspective

- Strong
- Kind
- Easy to get along with
- Hardworking
- Protector

PROFILE OF MRS. TAYLOR

From Her Perspective

- Basically conservative
- Has traditional belief
  systems
- Tries to live "the perfect
  family"
- Would like to find a job
  outside of the home
- Interested in music

From Randy's Perspective

- Gentle

- Organized
- Easy to talk with
- Understanding

From Mr. Taylor's
Perspective

- Smart household manager
- "Good" mother
- Very organized
- Friendly
- Helps everyone

From Jamie's Perspective

- Helpful
- Well-liked by friends
  and neighbors
- Generous
- Loving

PROFILE OF RANDY

From His Perspective

- Athletic
- Fun-loving
- Likes college
- Plans to be an engineer

From Mrs. Taylor's
Perspective

- Bright
- Has his own mind
- Likes sports

*From Mr. Taylor's
Perspective*

- "Good" student
- "He will turn out to be something"

From Jamie's Perspective

- "Makes me laugh"
- Easy to talk with
- "Helps me with math"
- Considerate
- Modest

PROFILE OF JAMIE

From Her Perspective

- Shy
- Not growing fast enough
- Sings in the church choir
- Likes to draw pictures of nature

*From Mrs. Taylor's
Perspective*

- Quiet
- Neat
- Intelligent

*From Mr. Taylor's
Perspective*

- Serious
- "Good" student
- Pretty

From Randy's Perspective

- Pleasant
- Thoughtful
- Talented

Decision-Making Pattern in the Taylor Family

Mr. and Mrs. Taylor discuss issues and come to a mutual agreement on major decisions. The children are becoming more and more a part of the family decision-making process. For example, the Taylors decided to purchase an automobile. All the members of the family participated in deciding the model and color.

Contextual Situation

As Mr. Taylor approached his doctor's office, he was annoyed and impatient as he thought about the work waiting for him at his office and the wasted time involved in this annual physical examination. He mused how his wife was much too concerned about these things and so organized that the visit was planned months ago. In Dr. Brown's office, however, his musing changed. Mr. Taylor's chest x-ray showed a shadow that could be a tumor, and perhaps a malignant one. Dr. Brown advised Mr. Taylor to be admitted at once to the hospital for more definitive studies. As he left the doctor's office, Mr. Taylor was aware of very different thoughts and perceptions. He was acutely aware of the potential meanings of the menacing spot; and, as this awareness unfolded for him, new insights and new values surfaced as he dwelled with the remembered and the imaged all at once. He could not help thinking about his wife and children as he confronted his non-being. The possibilities surfaced as he began to think

through how he would share with his family the information about the shadow on his lung. As he sat in
the park, he imaged telling them in many different
ways, no longer in a hurry to get to the office. Mr.
Taylor sat on a bench outside the medical complex and,
for the first time in a long time, knew the sunshine
on his face and the mild breeze through his hair. As
Mr. Taylor dwelled with one phenomena after the
other in his unfocused imaging, he connected and
separated all at once multidimensionally. He decided
to go home and discuss the matter with Mrs. Taylor
before the children arrived home for dinner. In sharing
the news with Mrs. Taylor, Mr. Taylor languaged his
pain as he sat slumped in the kitchen chair, unable to
drink the cup of tea he had requested. The two looked
at each other knowingly—both seeing in the other the
suffering. In coconstitution with each other, each
imaged possibilities. They came to know, in a new way,
their affection for each other and the children through
the surfacing of the non-being. The prized values of
future planning—a well-organized household and strict
rules—were viewed now with a different perspective
as Mr. and Mrs. Taylor revealed and concealed their
hopes and desires, fears and pain through their gestures,
facial expressions, and speech. As they began to discuss
the possibilities in the immediate and long-range future,
they uncovered the enabling and limiting aspects of the
event, as they struggled to integrate the unfamiliar
with the familiar. The ambiguity of the situation per-
meated the thoughts of Mr. and Mrs. Taylor as they
struggled to be more comfortable with the situation
and more certain about the future. They decided to
talk with the children about the situation and share
their concerns and the enabling-limiting possibilities.
On hearing the news, Jamie cried and hugged Mr.
Taylor. She said she was afraid. Her view of Mr. Taylor
as protector was brought into question as she con-

fronted the meaning of non-being for herself and for her father. Randy was quiet, not light-hearted, as he was confronted with the meaning of the event for him as the eldest child. He saw his father differently; for the first time he saw him as vulnerable, and this surfaced non-being for him. The Taylor family drew close together in struggling to transcend the paradoxes and create possibilities as the changing health priorities brought other viewpoints to the surface.

Discussion of Nursing Practice with the Taylor Family

Nursing practice for the Taylor family, based on the theory of Man-Living-Health, points to intersubjective participation in guiding them in the choosing of possibilities in the changing health process. A discussion follows relative to the focus of nursing practice for the Taylor family, in light of the theoretical structures posited in Chapter IV.

THEORETICAL STRUCTURE 1: POWERING IS A WAY OF REVEALING AND CONCEALING IMAGING

Nursing practice for the Taylor family, relative to this theoretical structure, focuses on illuminating the family's meaning, of the situation that is surfacing in the presence of the lung shadow. The focus is also on the process of revealing and concealing in illuminating the unique ways the family can mobilize energies to image new possibilities. The new possibilities move the family beyond the struggle of the immediate situation.

THEORETICAL STRUCTURE 2:
ORIGINATING IS A MANIFESTATION
OF ENABLING AND LIMITING VALUING

Nursing practice, relative to this theoretical structure, focuses on guiding the family in unfolding the prized values, particularly as related to living with the ambiguity of the situation. The focus is on illuminating the changing family values as members dwell with the enabling and limiting aspects of the situation for themselves as well as each other. The focus is also on mobilizing the family to reflectively change health priorities.

THEORETICAL STRUCTURE 3:
TRANSFORMING UNFOLDS IN THE
LANGUAGING OF CONNECTING
AND SEPARATING

Nursing practice, relative to this theoretical structure, focuses on guiding the Taylor family in choosing the particular change strategies with which the family is comfortable as the family languages meaning in connecting and separating in the situation. The focus is on illuminating the various perspectives each has of the others in the situation, as expressed in their languaging. The focus is also on mobilizing family energies toward integration of the unfamiliar, the newly surfacing meanings, with the familiar.

  The new discoveries that surface in nursing practice through intersubjective participation in guiding families in choosing possibilities in the changing health process will uncover research possibilities. When pursued, the research will enhance nursing's knowledge base.

IMPLICATIONS FOR EDUCATION

Man-Living-Health: A Theory of Nursing has implications for nursing education. Nursing curricula reflect current trends related to nursing's abstract body of knowledge. The purpose of nursing education programs is to transmit the body of nursing knowledge to those who will practice, teach, and do research in nursing. The curricula of baccalaureate, master's, and doctoral programs reflect this purpose. Doctoral programs in nursing, for example, focus on testing research methodologies, analyzing extant nursing theories, and developing nursing theory to prepare students to design and implement research studies which will enhance nursing's abstract body of knowledge. A curriculum based on the theoretical foundation of Man-Living-Health would be designed with a deliberate focus on the principles of this theory. First, emphasis would be placed on the philosophy of the program, and this philosophy would be present thematically throughout the structure of the curriculum. The concepts and theoretical structures of the theory of Man-Living-Health would be evident in all the elements of the curriculum: philosophy, program goals, program indicators, conceptual framework, themes, level and course indicators, course culture content, and evaluation process.

Elements of Curriculum

PROGRAM PHILOSOPHY AND GOALS

The philosophy of a school of nursing is a comprehensive statement of beliefs, representing the collective view of the entire faculty, about the relationship of man and health in the science and art of nursing. This statement of beliefs is arrived at through the ongoing process of negotiation as faculty members from diverse educational, social, and philosophical backgrounds come to an agreement on the basic underpinnings and unifying focus of a particular program. All other elements of the curriculum flow from the philosophy.

A philosophy includes a statement of specific beliefs about man, health, society, education, nursing's emerging role in society, and the teaching-learning process. These beliefs reflect, or should reflect, the general beliefs of the institution of which the school of nursing is a part. The program goals are broad aims that clearly reflect the intent of the program; they serve also, equally importantly, to guide the faculty, students, and administration in the educational process.

INDICATORS

Program indicators, when properly constructed, flow from the goals and specifically guide student learning toward optimum goal achievement. Indicators, like objectives, are beacons on which sights can be set in relation to goal achievement. Unlike objectives, however, indicators are far more general. While indicators always state specific content and action, they do not identify *exactly* how a student must perform to achieve a goal. The term *indicator* as used here is a far more open term than *objective* and explicitly reflects the subjective nature of all evaluative measures. Indicators strongly imply the responsibility of both the teacher and the learner in the evaluative process. They allow for deviation from the often abused and historically perpetuated myth that performance can be measured "objectively" by the teacher. When the philosophy of a school of nursing espouses the principle that evaluation of students is from the perspective of the teacher's worldview, the term *indicator* should be used instead of the term *objective* in order to promote and foster internal congruence in the overall curriculum design. The term *indicator*, then, is used in the design of a comprehensive curriculum plan whose theoretical underpinnings are based on a belief about man as a synergistic being cocreating an individual becoming.

Level indicators flow from the program goals and from the indicators. The level indicators identify the expected achievement in performance after the student has accrued a certain number of credit hours in a particular program. Each set of level indicators refers directly to a particular program goal and gives rise to the course goals and the indicators that are taught within that particular level. The course goals and indicators are the specific guides for student achievement in an individual course. The goals guide and focus the development of the course culture content. A synthesis of the course goals and indicators at a given level, then, are that level's indicators.

CONCEPTUAL FRAMEWORK AND THEMES

A conceptual framework, along with its support theories, flows clearly and directly from the philosophy and is the basic architectural blueprint from which the curriculum themes emerge; these themes, then, form the course culture content. The conceptual framework consists of the concepts that surface in the philosophy. The support theories are selected for their consistency with the beliefs outlined in the philosophy, and they complement the nursing theoretical base. The curriculum themes are the recurrent and ongoing patterns of ideas that unify all the courses within each level and all the courses from level to level.

COURSE CULTURE CONTENT

Course culture content refers to the specific conceptual focus of each separate unit of instruction. It reflects the conceptual framework, its support theories, and the entirety of its unifying themes, thus reflecting the philosophy of the program.

EVALUATION PROCESS

The evaluation plan for a program emerges from the philosophy and goals, as do all the other elements of the curriculum that have been discussed. Evaluation is a coconstituted process, one in which a value is given to growth toward a desired goal. An evaluation model, as well as methodologies, is constructed in congruence with the conceptual system of the program. Data that are collected in the comprehensive evaluation are interpreted, ordered, and used for decision making about the program. Methods used to obtain evaluation data are generally considered to be threefold; they are observation, interview, and survey. And there are five major elements to an evaluation system[3] : input, output, process, supplemental, and financial. *Input* refers to program precondition. Information gathered before entrance into the program establishes a baseline and includes data from the program pretest and from student profiles. The purpose of a program pretest is to ascertain the basic knowledge level of the students before they actually begin the program. When these data are later compared with posttest data, they demonstrate a dimension of what students have learned in the program. The profile includes information about student characteristics. The significant characteristics among these are age, sex, race, ethnic origin, marital status, educational background, significant work experience, Miller's Analogies results and Graduate Record Examination scores, scholarships and other academic honors, present work situation, nature of work, hours worked per week, academic references, professional references, and student status. *Output* refers to program outcome. Data are collected at varying specified points during the educational process, at the end of each course, at the end of each level, and at the end of the

[3] Richard M. Wolf, *Evaluation in Education* (New York: Praeger Publishers, Praeger Special Studies, 1979).

program. Information is gathered at the end of each course from the following two sources: (1) student self-evaluation and faculty evaluation of student performance, and (2) student evaluation of the overall conduct and impact of the course. Data gathered at each level end and at the end of the program denote student progress according to the goals and indicators. Faculty, independently and collectively, reflect on the performance of each student at each level and at the programs end and arrive at a decision on the performance by each student on each level indicator. These data are then compared with pretest data to determine student progress and the effectiveness of the program. *Process* refers to program execution. Data are collected in this instance to determine whether or not the various types of learning opportunities described in the program plan are being implemented in a satisfactory manner. The data are obtained from three different sources: (1) observation through class visitation; (2) inspection of course documents, student papers, bibliographies, student projects, and other related and ancillary materials; and (3) faculty and student evaluations about the course process. *Supplemental* refers to program impact. Data are collected from program faculty and students, families for whom the students provided service, and from the program graduates and their immediate supervisors in their place of employment. These data provide valuable information relative to perceptions of, reactions to, and opinions of the program among peer professionals in the nursing profession and the community at large. *Financial*, obviously, refers to program cost. The purpose of financial assessment is to determine the relative cost efficiency of the program. Data are collected in categories of both direct and indirect expenditures. Direct expenditures are instructional costs and program support costs. Indirect expenditures are instructional support costs and are sometimes difficult to identify clearly. Both direct and indirect expenditures are divided into basic and additional costs as well as into recurring and nonrecurring costs. The program financial evaluation plan, then, yields data on basic recurring costs, basic nonrecurring costs, additional recurring costs, and additional nonrecurring costs. The total amount of all costs is examined and evaluated in relation to the number of students in the program. Cost per student is then determined. The basic and additional recurring costs are used to project future costs of the program.

These five enumerated elements, then—input, output, process, supplemental, and financial—provide a clearly defined structure for a thorough and comprehensive assessment of a total program.

A Curriculum Plan Based on Man-Living-Health

Many different curricular patterns may be designed with the theory of Man-Living-Health as a theoretical base. The important factor in developing a curriculum plan, whatever its theoretical base, is that it has internal consistency. While the wording of one philosophy and the specific concepts in the conceptual framework would differ from that of another, the fundamental assumptions about man and health would be consistent and recognized throughout the plan. Following is a sample curriculum plan for a program leading to the degree, master of science in nursing. This plan is based on the principles, concepts, and theoretical structures of the theory of Man-Living-Health. The sample plan includes purpose, philosophy, conceptual framework, themes, program goals and indicators, level indicators, course sequence, descriptions, goals, some instructional and evaluation strategies for each course, and an evaluation plan.

SAMPLE PURPOSE OF THE PROGRAM

The purpose of the graduate program leading to a master of science degree in nursing is to provide a curriculum plan for guiding the learner in the achievement of certain goals, goals that will broaden the theoretical knowledge base of the learner in preparation for a leadership role and doctoral study. The nurse prepared at the master's level develops, tests, and evaluates concepts relevant for nursing and critically examines concepts and theories in relation to health issues, initiates nursing research, and practices nursing in a leadership role.

This master's program provides specialization in the area of family health and in two specific areas of role concentration: teaching nursing and administering nursing services. All students will be provided the opportunity to learn the theoretical base of Man-Living-Health and, consistent with this opportunity, will participate in practicum experiences with specially selected families. Those students selecting teaching nursing as their area of role concentration will be provided the opportunity to learn the theoretical base of the teaching-learning process from the perspective of Man-Living-Health. Practicum experiences for these students will be situated in baccalaureate level nursing programs. Those students selecting administering of nursing services as their area of role concentration will be provided with the opportunity to learn the theoretical base of the administrative process from the perspective of Man-Living-Health. Practicum experiences for these students will be situated in various health care agencies. The teacher of nursing who successfully completes this program has a specialization in family health and is prepared to assume a faculty position in a baccalaureate nursing program. The administrator of nursing services who graduates from this program is prepared to administer in a middle-management position in a health care system.

SAMPLE PHILOSOPHY OF THE PROGRAM

The faculty of the school of nursing believes that the academic discipline of nursing is a science and an art. It seeks to understand Man-Living-Health and provides a service to society through its concern for families' health care as well as their quality of living. Nursing focuses on guiding families in choosing possibilities in their changing health process. The nurse initiates interrelationships with families while illuminating with them their health patterns and mobilizing their energies for planned change. The nurse bases practice on the theory of Man-Living-Health. The nurse regularly conducts self-evaluations and plans for continuing self-enhancement. Through systematic inquiry, the nurse enhances the evolution of the nursing profession toward independence. Education for the leadership in nursing occurs in an institution of higher learning granting master's and doctoral degrees in nursing. Teacher and learner coconstitute the educational process through sharing knowledge and planning educationally sound and fulfilling experiences. Ideas are investigated regularly and systematically in an effort to uncover new knowledge.

The philosophical tenets that underpin this graduate nursing program are the assumptions about man and health from which the theory of Man-Living-Health evolves. These assumptions are as follows:

- Man is coexisting while coconstituting rhythmical patterns with the environment.
- Man is an open being, freely choosing meaning in situation, bearing responsibility for decisions.
- Man is a living unity continuously coconstituting patterns of relating.

- Man is transcending multidimensionally with the possibles.
- Health is an open process of becoming, experienced by man.
- Health is a rhythmically coconstituting process of the man-environment interrelationship.
- Health is man's patterns of relating value priorities.
- Health is an intersubjective process of transcending with the possibles.
- Health is unitary man's negentropic unfolding.

For this program, then, Man-Living-Health is a unifying phenomenon expressing man's unique way of being with the world. Man-Living-Health is man's becoming. Man's becoming is a unitary process of negentropically unfolding as man chooses health possibilities. These possibilities emerge in the process of family interrelationships. Through these interrelationships meaning is given to events as man coconstitutes situations through the languaging of imaged values. Man-Living-Health is an expression of values freely chosen in situation. Man-Living-Health is cocreating rhythmical patterns of relating. These patterns of relating are the recognizable features that identify man as an individual living in coexistence with others. Man-Living-Health is an expression of the open energy interchange between man and environment in the process of becoming. Living health is powering transformation through a personal originating of meaning and changing in situation. The meaning and changing surface for each person in a unique way relative to that person's historicity involving belief systems that span decades or more and that arise from generational and multicultural society. Families and health-care promoters, being aware of these same belief systems, participate in mobilizing energies for change. The graduate nursing program in this school of nursing builds on baccalaureate education and prepares specialists in family health with an area of role concentration in either teaching nursing or administering nursing services. The graduate nursing program emphasizes and concentrates on concept development, that is, the creating and testing of concepts. Also highlighted are theoretical foundations of leadership and rigorous inquiry in research. The program is directed mainly toward the evolution and testing of nursing theory, and it illuminates clearly the interrelationship of theory, practice, research, and education.

SAMPLE CONCEPTUAL FRAMEWORK OF THE PROGRAM

The conceptual framework emerges quite naturally from the philosophy. There are five concepts delineated in the philosophy, and they form the conceptual framework of this program. These are negentropic unfolding, choosing meaning, patterns of relating, synergistic becoming, and personal originating. The major unifying themes emerging from these seminal concepts are valuing, transforming, cocreating, and powering. Schema 9 depicts the concepts, themes, support theories, and theorists from whom to draw relative to the concepts and themes emerging from the philosophy.

SAMPLE PROGRAM GOALS AND INDICATORS OF THE PROGRAM

In this program students and faculty coconstitute the teaching-learning process. Students are encouraged throughout to be self-directive. Each student, with the assistance of faculty members, is expected to identify personal goals consistent with the program goals, plan meaningful experiences, and evaluate the achievement of goals. Program evaluation is a continuous process shared between and among students,

SCHEMA 9. SAMPLE CONCEPTUAL FRAMEWORK, THEMES, SUPPORT THEORIES, AND THEORISTS

Program focus:	Leadership. inquiry
Theoretical base:	The theory of Man-Living-Health
Nurse theorist:	Parse

Concepts	Unifying Themes
Negentropic unfolding	Valuing
Choosing meaning	Transforming
Patterns of relating	Cocreating
Synergistic becoming	Powering
Personal originating	

Support Theories	Theorists
Change theory	J. H. van den Berg
	P. Watzlawick
Teaching-learning theory	J. Dewey
	M. Greene
	C. Rogers
Leadership theory	R. Burns
	P. Drucker
Family theory	W. Kempler
Research theory	A. Kaplan
	F. Kerlinger
	H. Spiegelburg

faculty, and consumers. The program goals and indicators are as follows:

GOAL 1:

To practice, in a leadership role, nursing based on the theory of Man-Living-Health.

INDICATORS:

- Understands concepts related to Man-Living-Health.
- Guides families in choosing possibilities in their changing health process.
- Demonstrates self-direction.

- Demonstrates accountability to families.
- Initiates collaborative relationships with families and peer professionals.

GOAL 2:

To practice a leadership role of teaching nursing or administering nursing services from the theoretical base of Man-Living-Health.

INDICATORS:

- Promotes the delivery of quality health care through teaching nursing or administering nursing services.
- Promotes change in social systems based on the theoretical perspective of Man-Living-Health.
- Teaches nursing or administers nursing services from the theoretical base of Man-Living-Health.
- Compares value priorities in decision making.
- Demonstrates accountability to self and peer professionals.

GOAL 3:

To utilize the process of inquiry.

INDICATORS:

- Uses a systematic method of study in nursing.
- Uses research findings to enhance decision making.
- Tests the theory of Man-Living-Health.
- Compares various perspectives as part of decision making.
- Makes judgments based on a theoretical perspective.
- Specifies value priorities in decision making.

GOAL 4:

To contribute to theory evolution in nursing.

INDICATORS:

- Develops concepts from the perspective of Man-Living-Health relevant for nursing.
- Validates concepts for their applicability to the theory of Man-Living-Health.

SAMPLE LEVEL INDICATORS
FOR THE PROGRAM

There are two levels identified in this graduate nursing program. Level I evaluation occurs after completion of the first 24 credits and level II evaluation after completion of 48 total credits in the program.

Student progress is evaluated at Levels I and II in accordance with specific indicators. A satisfactory performance for all indicators at each of the two evaluation points is required.

PROGRAM GOAL I:

To practice in a leadership role nursing based on the theory of Man-Living-Health.

LEVEL I INDICATORS (evaluation after 24 credits):

- Comprehends concepts related to Man-Living-Health.
- Illuminates patterns of relating with families.
- Demonstrates self-direction.
- Demonstrates accountability to families.
- Initiates collaborative relationships with families and peer professionals.

LEVEL II INDICATORS (evaluation after 48 credits):

- Understands concepts related to Man-Living-Health.
- Guides families in choosing possibilities in their changing health process.
- Demonstrates self-direction.

- Demonstrates accountability to families.
- Initiates collaborative relationships with families and peer professionals.

PROGRAM GOAL II:
To practice a leadership role of teaching nursing or administering nursing services from the theoretical base of Man-Living-Health.

LEVEL I INDICATORS (evaluation after 24 credits):
- Identifies quality health care from the perspective of Man-Living-Health.
- Identifies change strategies related to theoretical perspectives.
- Incorporates principles of teaching or administration with the theory of Man-Living-Health.
- Compares value priorities relative to nursing issues.
- Demonstrates accountability to self and peer professionals.

LEVEL II INDICATORS (evaluation after 48 credits):
- Promotes the delivery of quality health care through teaching nursing or administering nursing services.
- Promotes change in social systems based on the theoretical perspective of Man-Living-Health.
- Teaches nursing or administers nursing services from the theoretical base of Man-Living-Health.
- Compares value priorities in decision making.
- Demonstrates accountability to self and peer professionals.

PROGRAM GOAL III:
To utilize the process of inquiry.

LEVEL I INDICATORS (evaluation after 24 credits):
- Uses a systematic method to study concepts of Man-Living-Health.

- Uses literature to support conclusions.
- Comprehends the elements of the theory of Man-Living-Health.
- Examines various perspectives related to nursing issues.
- Identifies judgments as based on theoretical foundations.
- Delineates value priorities in qualifying convictions.

LEVEL II INDICATORS (evaluation after 48 credits):
- Uses a systematic method of study in nursing.
- Uses research findings to enhance decision making.
- Tests the theory of Man-Living-Health.
- Compares various perspectives as part of decision making.
- Makes judgments based on a theoretical perspective.
- Specifies value priorities in decision making.

PROGRAM GOAL IV:
To contribute to theory evolution in nursing.

LEVEL I INDICATORS (evaluation after 24 credits):
- Develops concepts from the perspective of Man-Living-Health relevant for nursing.
- Compares extant nursing theories.

LEVEL II INDICATORS (evaluation after 48 credits):
- Develops concepts from the perspective of Man-Living-Health relevant for nursing.
- Validates concepts for their applicability to the theory of Man-Living-Health.

SAMPLE COURSE PLAN

The focus of the courses in this curriculum design is on advanced knowledge and practice of nursing science. The courses evolve from the level indicators. The course design has three structural components: focal courses, subsidiary courses, and role courses.

Focal Courses

There are five three-credit courses that provide an opportunity for in-depth study of nursing science, concept development and theory evolution, inquiry, leadership, and family. All these courses are didactic. The focal courses in the curriculum, with their module titles, are

Nursing Science: Man-Living-Health: Assumptions about man and health; principles, concepts, and theoretical structures of the theory

Concept Development and Theory Evolution: The construction of the theory of Man-Living-Health; extant theories and theory evolution.

Leadership Foundations: Change, valuing, and learning; change, valuing, and decision making; change, valuing; and evaluation

Nursing Research I: Experimental research designs; descriptive research designs

Family: Family process, issues, contextual grounding, and themes

Subsidiary Courses

A series of six three-credit courses provides in-depth study of leadership, inquiry, and concept development in family-nurse process. Five of these courses have nursing practice components and are both didactic and practicum in nature. The didactic dimension of these courses provides learning opportunities in three areas: inquiry, concept development, and leadership. The practicum dimension of these courses provides learning opportunities in testing concepts through family-nurse process. Practicum time is spent with families in individual consultation with faculty and in peer review seminars. One of these courses in an independent research project that provides learning opportunities in validating concepts through a pilot study. The subsidiary courses in this curriculum, with their module titles, are

Family-Nurse Process I: Languaging and family health; powering health possibilities

Family-Nurse Process II: Evolutionary and planned change; continuity of change

Family-Nurse Process III: Health myths and metaphors; multicultural transformation

Family Patterns of Relating: Struggle and commitment in family-nurse process; cocreating synergistic becoming

Family Life Experiences: Personal originating and family life experiences; caring as a function of healing

Nursing Research II: Independent research project

Role Courses

There are five three-credit courses in the role concentration areas of teaching nursing and administering nursing services. These courses provide an opportunity for indepth study in inquiry, leadership, and concept testing. Two of these five courses are required courses in each of the role areas. Of these two, one in each area is didactic and the other has both didactic and practicum components. The didactic courses provide learning opportunities related to curriculum process in the teaching role area and administrative process in the administering of nursing services role area. The courses with both a didactic and a practicum dimension provide opportunities to study and test concepts in a leadership role. These courses and module titles follow:

Teaching Nursing Role Area

Curriculum Process: Curriculum development process; curriculum plan

Teaching Nursing Practicum: Teaching nursing model; responsibilities inherent in being a teacher of nursing

Administering Nursing Role Area

Administrative Process: Structure of administrative process; administrative plan

Administering Nursing Practicum: Administering nursing services model; responsibilities inherent in being a nurse administrator

Electives

Three of the five role courses are electives. These courses are didactic and provide an opportunity for students to choose three from five possible options. The electives embellish aspects of the role areas and encourage in-depth study in the topics offered. The five elective options in the curriculum, with their module titles, are

Political Issues in Nursing Leadership: Participation in health policy making; legal-ethical-moral responsibilities in nursing leadership roles

Nursing Leadership and Technological Resources: Science and technology; utilization of technological resources in leadership situations

Comparative Studies in Nursing Leadership: Education and administration in the People's Republic of China; education and administration in the Soviet Union

Nursing Leadership and Health Care Systems: Peer professional relationships; change strategies in a multicultural system

Nursing Leadership and Institutions of Higher Learning: Academic disciplines; change strategies in academia

SAMPLE COURSE SEQUENCE

The graduate program leading to a master of science degree in nursing may be obtained through completion of a curriculum plan. This program may be completed on a full- or part-time basis. The program is 48 credits in length.

FULL-TIME COURSE SEQUENCE

Fall Semester	Cr	Spring Semester	Cr
Nursing Science: Man-Living-Health	3	Family-Nurse Process I	3
Concept Development and Theory Evolution	3	Curriculum or Administrative Process	3
		Role Elective	3
Leadership Foundations	3	Family Life Experiences	3
Family	3		
	12		12

Fall Semester	Cr	Spring Semester	Cr
Nursing Research I	3	Nursing Research II	3
Family-Nurse Process II	3	Family-Nurse Process III	3
Role Elective	3	Teaching Nursing or Administering Nursing Practicum	3
Family Patterns of Relating	3	Role Elective	3
	12		12

PART-TIME COURSE SEQUENCE

Fall Semester	Cr	Spring Semester	Cr
Nursing Science: Man-Living-Health	3	Curriculum or Administrative Process	3
Concept Development and Theory Evolution	3	Role Elective	3
	6		6

Fall Semester	Cr	*Spring Semester*	Cr
Leadership Foundations	3	Family-Nurse Process I	3
Family	3	Family Life Experiences	3
	6		6

Fall Semester	Cr	*Spring Semester*	Cr
Family-Nurse Process II	3	Family-Nurse Process III	3
Family Patterns of Relating	3	Role Elective	3
	6		6

Fall Semester	Cr	*Spring Semester*	Cr
Role Elective	3	Teaching Nursing or Administering Nursing Practicum	3
Nursing Research I	3	Nursing Research II	3
	6		6

SAMPLE INSTRUCTIONAL STRATEGIES

Some instructional strategies used in this graduate nursing program would be faculty-student process, family-nurse process, student-student process, teacher-student process, administrator-nurse process, and student-group process.

Faculty-student process is the interrelationship that evolves between teacher and student. Faculty and student collaborate from initial curriculum planning throughout the educational experience. Faculty guide students in one-to-one relationships and in small groups in each course in the graduate nursing program.

Family-nurse process is an instructional strategy that entails an evolving interrelationship between family and nursing student. In each subsidiary course, students are required to test concepts related to Man-

Living-Health through family-nurse process. Testing concepts in the family-nurse process entails illuminating and mobilizing family energies toward changing health patterns. Testing and evaluating is done by recording the family-nurse process on videotape. This recording is analyzed by student and faculty for the purpose of student evaluation. The videotape, as a mechanism supporting this instructional strategy, allows the student to view the family-nurse process as a data base for concept development.

Student-student process is the interrelationship evolving among students as they develop peer professional relationships. Peer collaboration and evaluation is encouraged through small-group projects and peer review sessions related to family-nurse process, teacher-student process, and administrator-nurse process. Students share the opportunity to interrogate and test concepts in the process of concept development, inquiry, and leadership. All subsidiary and role courses use student-student process as an instructional strategy.

Teacher-student process is an instructional strategy for all students in the teaching role area. Each student teacher of nursing creates a teaching model that is tested in a teaching situation. The testing of the model entails communication with baccalaureate students. Interrelationships between the student teacher of nursing and baccalaureate nursing students is videotaped for analysis and evaluation.

Administrator-nurse process is an instructional strategy for all students participating in the administering of nursing services role area. The student administrator of nursing services creates an administration model that is tested in a health-care system. The testing of the model entails communication with staff nurses. Interrelationships between the student administrator of nursing services and staff nurses is videotaped for analysis and evaluation.

Student-group process is an instructional strategy

that encourages the student to develop skill in planning and organizing toward goals. It further gives students the opportunity to guide group process toward a goal. Some student-group process sessions are videotaped for analysis and evaluation. Student-group process is used in all courses. These instructional strategies are samples of those that would be used in a graduate nursing program whose theoretical base is Man-Living-Health.

SAMPLE COURSE DESCRIPTIONS, GOALS, INDICATORS, CONCEPTUAL FOCUS, INSTRUCTIONAL AND EVALUATION STRATEGIES

Following are sample course descriptions, goals, indicators, the conceptual focus and goals of each module, and some instructional and evaluation strategies for each course in the sample curriculum plan. The course culture content that is explicitly articulated in the course descriptions and goals evolves from the level indicators and reflects the conceptual framework and unifying themes in the philosophy.

Focal Courses

The focal courses provide a foundation in theory development, inquiry, and leadership upon which the subsidiary and role courses build. These five courses are three credits each and didactic.

Course Title: Nursing Science: Man-Living-Health

Course Description: This course provides an opportunity to study the assumptions about man and health underpinning the theory of Man-Living-Health. It emphasizes the principles, concepts, and theoretical structures of the theory. Participants are invited to examine these systematically and appropriate the theory. Participants are further invited to relate the meaning of the theory to nursing practice.

Goals and Indicators:

To utilize the process of inquiry.

- Examines systematically the elements of the theory of Man-Living-Health.
- Uses literature to support convictions.
- Delineates value priorities in qualifying convictions.
- Demonstrates self-direction in studying Man-Living-Health.

To understand the assumptions underpinning the theory of Man-Living-Health.

- Examines the concepts synthesized in each assumption.
- Compares the meaning of each assumption.
- Synthesizes the meaning of the assumptions as a basis for nursing practice.

To comprehend the theory of Man-Living-Health.

- Examines the principles, concepts, and theoretical structures of Man-Living-Health.
- Relates each principle to the basic assumptions of the theory.
- Relates the theoretical structures to nursing practice.

Conceptual Focus:

Module I: Assumptions about Man and Health
Goals: To utilize the process of inquiry.

	To understand the assumptions underpinning the theory of Man-Living-Health.
Module II:	Principles, Concepts, and Theoretical Structures of Man-Living-Health.
Goals:	To utilize the process of inquiry.
	To comprehend the theory of Man-Living-Health.

Instructional Strategies:

Faculty-student process

Student-group process

Evaluation: Evaluation is based on achievement of the goals of the course as evidenced by

- Performance as group leader
- Quality of two papers
- Performance on final examination

■

Course Title: Concept Development and Theory Evolution

Course Description: This course provides an opportunity to study concept and theory building in nursing. Emphasis is placed on the process of building the theory of Man-Living-Health. Participants are invited to examine and analyze the elements of the theory of Man-Living-Health as well as other extant theories. Participants are further invited to create a concept congruent with the theory of Man-Living-Health and propose testing for applicability to nursing.

Goals and Indicators:

To utilize the process of inquiry.

- Uses a systematic method to study theory evolution.

- Uses appropriate literature to support concept development.
- Delineates value priorities in creating an original concept.
- Demonstrates self-direction in studying concept development and theory evolution.

To understand the process of theory construction.

- Examines the elements of a theory.
- Compares extant nursing theories.
- Comprehends the elements of the theory of Man-Living-Health.

To contribute to concept development.

- Develops an original concept congruent with the theory of Man-Living-Health.
- Tests the applicability of the concept for nursing.

Conceptual Focus:

Module I: The Construction of the Theory of Man-Living-Health.

Goals: To utilize the process of inquiry.

To understand the process of theory construction.

Module II: Extant Nursing Theories and Theory Evolution.

Goals: To utilize the process of inquiry.

To contribute to concept development.

Instructional Strategies:

Faculty-student process

Student-group process

Group project related to extant theories

Evaluation: Evaluation is based on achievement of the goals of the course as evidenced by

- Performance as group leader
- Quality of project
- Quality of two papers
- Performance on final examination

■

Course Title: Leadership Foundations

Course Description: This course provides an opportunity to study the theoretical basis for the leadership roles of nursing teacher and nursing administrator. It emphasizes valuing and change as related to the processess of learning, decision-making, and evaluation. Participants are invited to examine and test concepts and theories related to change, valuing, learning, decision making, and evaluation and to synthesize these into a conceptual framework for leadership congruent with the theory of Man-Living-Health.

Goals and Indicators:

To utilize the process of inquiry.

- Uses a systematic method to study the processes of leadership.
- Uses appropriate literature to validate conclusions.
- Delineates value priorities related to leadership.
- Demonstrates self-direction in studying leadership concepts.
- Identifies judgments based on theoretical foundations.

To synthesize the concepts of change, valuing, and learning with the theory of Man-Living-Health.

- Examines concepts and theories of learning related to the leadership process.
- Integrates learning concepts with the theory of Man-Living-Health.
- Compares value priorites in relation to change and learning.
- Identifies change strategies related to learning.

To synthesize the concepts of change, valuing, and decision making with the theory of Man-Living-Health.

- Examines concepts and theories of decision making related to the leadership process.
- Integrates decision-making concepts with the theory of Man-Living-Health.
- Compares value priorities in relation to change and decision making.
- Identifies change strategies related to decision making.

To synthesize the concepts of change, valuing, and evaluation with the theory of Man-Living-Health.

- Examines concepts and theories of evaluation related to the leadership process.
- Integrates evaluation concepts with the theory of Man-Living-Health.
- Compares value priorities in relation to change and evaluation.
- Identifies change strategies related to evaluation.

Conceptual Focus:

Module I: Change, Valuing, and Learning
Goals: To utilize the process of inquiry.
             To synthesize the concepts of change,

valuing, and learning with the theory of Man-Living-Health.

Module II: Change, Valuing, and Decision Making.

Goals: To utilize the process of inquiry.

To synthesize the concepts of change, valuing, and decision making with the theory of Man-Living-Health.

Module III: Change, Valuing, and Evaluation

Goals: To utilize the process of inquiry.

To synthesize concepts of change, valuing, and evaluation with the theory of Man-Living-Health.

Instructional Strategies:

Faculty-student process

Student-group process

Individual leadership project

Evaluation: Evaluation is based on achievement of the goals of the course as evidenced by

- Performance as group leader
- Quality of leadership project
- Quality of two papers
- Performance on final examination

■

Course Title: Nursing Research I

Course Description: This course provides an opportunity to study the research process in depth primarily as it relates to verification of the theory of Man-Living-Health. It emphasizes the systematic examination of experimental and descriptive research designs. Participants are invited to develop a research proposal using a descriptive methodology related to verifying the theory of Man-Living-Health.

Goals and Indicators:

To utilize the process of inquiry.

- Uses a systematic method to study research and design.
- Uses appropriate literature to validate conclusions.
- Demonstrates self-direction in studying research design.
- Delineates value priorities in studying research design.

To understand the theoretical basis of experimental research designs.

- Identifies the elements of experimental research designs.
- Analyzes nursing research studies using natural science research criteria.

To understand the theoretical basis of descriptive research designs.

- Identifies the descriptive research methodologies.
- Develops research questions relevant to nursing.
- Develops a research proposal related to verifying the theory of Man-Living-Health.

Conceptual Focus:

Module I: Experimental Research Designs

Goals: To utilize the process of inquiry.

To understand the theoretical basis of experimental research designs.

Module II: Descriptive Research Designs

Goals: To utilize the process of inquiry.

To understand the theoretical basis of descriptive research designs.

Instructional Strategies:
  Faculty-student process
  Research proposal

Evaluation: Evaluation is based on achievement of the
goals of the course as evidenced by

- Quality of research proposal
- Performance on final examination

■

Course Title: Family

Course Description: This course provides an opportunity to study family theories and family issues, contextual grounding, and themes. It emphasizes the
various theoretical perspectives of family systems and
structure as they relate to choosing meaning and
negentropic unfolding. Participants are invited to
examine these various theoretical perspectives in
relation to the theory of Man-Living-Health. Participants are further invited to examine several family
issues and the contextual grounding and themes
that emerge in family process.

Goals and Indicators:
  To utilize the process of inquiry.

- Uses a systematic method of examining family
  theories.
- Uses appropriate literature to support conclusions.
- Demonstrates self-direction in studying family.
- Delineates value priorities in qualifying convictions.

To understand family from various theoretical perspectives.

- Examines family process from the theoretical

perspectives of systems and structure as related to choosing meaning and negentropic unfolding.
- Synthesizes concepts of family with the theory of Man-Living-Health.

To understand family issues, contextual grounding, and emergent themes in family process.

- Examines family process from the perspective of Man-Living-Health.
- Examines issues in family process.
- Compares contextual grounding and emergent themes in family process. ‸

Conceptual Focus:
  Module I: Family Process
  Goals: To utilize the process of inquiry.
             To understand family from various theoretical perspectives.
  Module II: Family Issues, Contextual Grounding, and Themes
  Goals: To utilize the process of inquiry.
             To understand family issues, contextual grounding, and emergent themes in family process.

Instructional Strategies:
  Faculty-student process
  Student-group process
  Family-related project

Evaluation: Evaluation is based on achievement of the goals of the course as evidenced by:

- Performance as group leader
- Quality of two papers

- Quality of family-related project
- Performance on final examination

Subsidiary Courses

The subsidiary courses are built on the foundation of focal courses. They build on theory development, inquiry, and leadership in family-nurse process and research process. These courses have didactic and practicum components and are three credits each. Didactic is one and one-half credits and practicum one and one-half credits. On a 2:1 ratio, one and one-half hours of didactic and three hours of practicum are required each week. One course focuses on the research process and is completed on an independent study basis. The course descriptions, goals, indicators, conceptual focus and goals of each module, and some instructional and evaluation strategies for each of the subsidiary courses follow.

Course Title: Family-Nurse Process I

Course Description: This course provides an opportunity to study family process in depth. It emphasizes the creation of a conceptual framework for the testing of the theory of Man-Living-Health with families. Participants are invited to select at least four families with whom to study family languaging and the powering of health possibilities through family process.

Goals and Indicators:

To utilize the process of inquiry.

- Uses a systematic method of inquiry to study family-nurse process.
- Uses appropriate literature to substantiate decision making.
- Demonstrates self-direction in family-nurse process.

- Delineates value priorities in selection of families.
- Demonstrates accountability to families.

To test the relationship of family languaging to family health in family-nurse process.

- Illuminates language patterns with family as they relate to health.
- Initiates collaborative relationships with families.
- Recognizes own patterns of relating with families.
- Mobilizes family energies toward changing family health through languaging.

To test the concept of powering health possibilities in family-nurse process.

- Uncovers health possibilities with families.
- Mobilizes family energies toward planned goals.

Conceptual Focus:
    Module I: Languaging and Family Health
    Goals: To utilize the process of inquiry.
                 To test the relationship of family languaging to family health in family-nurse process.
    Module II: Powering Health Possibilities
    Goals: To utilize the process of inquiry.
                 To test the concept of powering health possibilities in family-nurse process.

Instructional Strategies:
  Faculty-student process
  Family-nurse process
  Student-student process
  Student-group process

Evaluation: Evaluation is based on the achievement of the goals of the course as evidenced by:

- Performance as group leader
- Quality of two papers
- Family-nurse process analyses
- Performance on final examination
- Performance in peer review

■

Course Title: Family-Nurse Process II

Course Description: This course builds on Family-Nurse Process I and provides an opportunity to study change and family process. It emphasizes concepts and theories related to evolutionary and planned change as well as the meaning of the continuity of change for family process. Participants are invited to test the theory of Man-Living-Health as it relates to change in the family health process. Participants are further invited to select at least one family with whom to study change in family health patterns over a period of time. Learning opportunities encourage testing and evaluation of change strategies for nursing practice, theory development, and research.

Goals and Indicators:

To utilize the process of inquiry.

- Uses a systematic method of inquiry to study change in family process.
- Uses appropriate literature to substantiate family change strategies.
- Demonstrates self-direction in the family-nurse process related to family change.
- Demonstrates accountability to families.

To implement change strategies through family-nurse process.

- Initiates collaborative relationships with families.
- Identifies with family strategies for health pattern changes.
- Mobilizes family energies toward planned change.

To evaluate change strategies in family-nurse process.

- Analyzes the continuity of change in family health process.
- Develops criteria with family to assess effectiveness of change strategies.
- Assesses change strategies related to family health patterns.

Conceptual Focus:

Module I: Evolutionary and Planned Change
Goals: To utilize the process of inquiry.
To implement change strategies through family-nurse process.
Module II: Continuity of Change
Goals: To utilize the process of inquiry.
To evaluate change strategies in family-nurse process.

Instructional Strategies:

Faculty-student process
Family-nurse process
Student-student process
Student-group process

Evaluation: Evaluation is based on the achievement of the goals of the course as evidenced by:

- Performance as group leader
- Quality of two papers
- Family-nurse process analyses
- Performance on final examination
- Performance in peer review

■

Course Title: Family-Nurse Process III

Course Description: This course builds on Family-Nurse Process II and provides an opportunity to study transformation in generational family process. It emphasizes concepts and theories related to the health myths and metaphors in multicultural family transformations. Participants are invited to test the theory of Man-Living-Health with generational families from a variety of cultures. Participants are further invited to select at least two families with whom to study negentropic unfolding through multicultural health myths and metaphors. Learning opportunities encourage testing and evaluation of these concepts for nursing practice, theory development, and research.

Goals and Indicators:

To utilize the process of inquiry.

- Uses a systematic method to study myths and metaphors in multicultural transformation.
- Uses appropriate literature to substantiate decision making in family-nurse process.
- Demonstrates self-direction in studying negentropic unfolding in family-nurse process.
- Demonstrates accountability to families.

To test the relationship of myths and metaphors to family health.

- Analyzes myths and metaphors in relation to family health patterns.
- Illuminates health myths and metaphors with families in the family-nurse process.
- Mobilizes family energies toward change in relation to family myths and metaphors.

To test the theory of Man-Living-Health with multicultural families.

- Understands concepts related to Man-Living-Health.
- Initiates collaborative relationships with families and peer professionals.
- Guides the family in choosing possibilities in the changing health process.
- Illuminates with family the multicultural transformation process.
- Mobilizes family energies toward planned transformation.

Conceptual Focus:

Module I: Health Myths and Metaphors
Goals: To utilize the process of inquiry.
           To test the relationship of myths and metaphors to family health.
Module II: Multicultural Transformation
Goals: To utilize the process of inquiry.
           To test the theory of Man-Living-Health with multicultural families.

Instructional Strategies:

Faculty-student process
Family-nurse process
Student-student process

Student-group process
Multicultural family project

Evaluation: Evaluation is based on the achievement of
the goals of the course as evidenced by:

- Performance as group leader
- Quality of two papers
- Family-nurse process analyses
- Quality of multicultural family project
- Performance on final examination
- Performance in peer review

■

Course Title: Family Patterns of Relating

Course Description: This course provides an opportunity to study family patterns of relating with the
concepts of commitment and struggle. It emphasizes
the rhythms of enabling-limiting, revealing-concealing,
and connecting-separating in family-nurse process.
Participants are invited to test these patterns of
relating as the basis of synergistic becoming with at
least two families.

Goals and Indicators:

To utilize the process of inquiry.

- Uses a systematic method to study family health
  patterns.
- Uses appropriate literature to support conclusions.
- Demonstrates self-direction in studying family
  health patterns.
- Delineates value priorities related to family health
  patterns.
- Demonstrates accountability to families.

To test the theory of Man-Living-Health in relationship to struggle and commitment in family-nurse process.

- Initiates collaborative relationships with families.
- Illuminates the meaning of struggle and commitment in family-nurse process.
- Mobilizes family energies toward struggle in commitment.

To test the relationship of patterns of relating to synergistic family becoming.

- Illuminates patterns of relating with families.
- Illuminates with families the meaning of synergistic becoming.
- Mobilizes family energies toward change in patterns of relating.

Conceptual Focus:

Module I: Struggle and Commitment in Family-Nurse Process

Goals: To utilize the process of inquiry.

To test the theory of Man-Living-Health in relationship to struggle and commitment in family-nurse process.

Module II: Cocreating Synergistic Becoming

Goals: To utilize the process of inquiry.

To test the relationship of patterns of relating to synergistic family becoming.

Instructional Strategies:

Faculty-student process

Family-nurse process

Student-student process

Student-group process

Evaluation: Evaluation is based on the achievement of the goals of the course as evidenced by:

- Performance as group leader
- Quality of two papers
- Performance on final examination
- Performance in peer review

■

Course Title: Family Life Experiences

Course Description: This course provides an opportunity to study some inevitable family life experiences. It emphasizes personal originating through birthing, dying, ambiguity, mystery, caring, and healing in the family health process. Participants are invited to test these concepts with families from the perspective of the theory of Man-Living-Health. Participants are invited to select at least two families with whom to study these inevitable family life experiences.

Goals and Indicators:

To utilize the process of inquiry.

- Uses a systematic method to study inevitable family life experiences.
- Uses appropriate literature to support conclusions.
- Demonstrates self-direction in studying family life experiences.
- Demonstrates accountability to families.
- Delineates value priorities in studying family life experiences.

To test the concept of personal originating as it relates to inevitable family life experiences.

- Integrates the meaning of personal originating

with the concepts of birthing, dying, ambiguity, and mystery.

- Illuminates the idea of personal originating through family-nurse process.
- Mobilizes family energies toward reflective originating in birthing the moment and in living with ambiguity.

To test family caring as a function of healing from the perspective of Man-Living-Health.

- Initiates collaborative relationships with families.
- Illuminates caring patterns in family-nurse process.
- Mobilizes family energies relative to healing in the caring process.

Conceptual Focus:

Module I: Personal Originating and Family Life Experiences

Goals: To utilize the process of inquiry.

To test the concept of personal originating as it relates to inevitable family life experiences.

Module II: Family Caring as a Function of Healing

Goals: To utilize the process of inquiry.

To test family caring as a function of healing from the perspective of Man-Living-Health.

Instructional Strategies:

Faculty-student process

Family-nurse process

Student-student process

Student-group process

Evaluation: Evaluation is based on the achievement of the goals of the course as evidenced by:

- Performance as group leader
- Quality of two papers
- Performance on final examination
- Performance in peer review

■

Course Title: Nursing Research II

Course Description: This course provides an opportunity to verify the theory of Man-Living-Health by implementing the descriptive research proposal designed in Nursing Research I. It emphasizes the implementation of a pilot study of an original concept.

Goals and Indicators:

To utilize the process of inquiry.

- Uses the appropriate systematic method of study in implementing research.
- Uses research findings to enhance decision making.
- Demonstrates self-direction in implementing a pilot study.

To implement a pilot study to verify the theory of Man-Living-Health.

- Protects the rights of research participants.
- Tests the theory of Man-Living-Health.
- Analyzes the research data according to the research design.
- Unfolds a general structure of the lived experience being studied.
- Proposes ideas for further study.

Instructional and Evaluation Strategies: This course is offered on an independent study basis. Faculty-student process predominates as the instructional strategy. A pass or fail grade is earned by the student. The evaluation is based on the quality of the pilot study report, which is the master's thesis for this graduate program.

Role Courses

The role courses build on the focal courses and enhance the subsidiary courses in the areas of theory development, inquiry, and leadership. Of the five role courses, two are required. Both are three credits. One is didactic; the other has a practicum component. The course with the practicum dimension is one credit of didactic and two credits of practicum. One hour of didactic and four hours of practicum are required each week. The other three courses are three-credit didactic electives. The course descriptions, goals, indicators, conceptual focus and goals of each module, and some instructional and evaluation strategies for each of the role courses follows.

TEACHING NURSING ROLE AREA:
REQUIRED COURSES

Course Title: Curriculum Process
Course Description: This course provides an opportunity to study concepts and theories related to curriculum development from a variety of conceptual perspectives. It emphasizes the elements of curriculum process. Participants are invited to design a curriculum plan from the perspective of Man-Living-Health for a baccalaureate nursing program. The plan includes philosophy, goals, indicators, level indicators, conceptual framework, themes, course culture content, course

sequence, instructional strategies, and an evaluation plan.

Goals and Indicators:

To utilize the process of inquiry.

- Uses a systematic method to study concepts and theories related to curriculum development.
- Uses research findings to validate curriculum planning.
- Demonstrates self-direction in studying the curriculum process.
- Specifies value priorities in decision making related to the curriculum process.
- Compares various perspectives as part of decision making in the curriculum process.
- Demonstrates accountability to self and peer professionals.

To understand the curriculum process.

- Analyzes curriculum theory from various perspectives.
- Critically examines the interpersonal process related to curriculum development.

To utilize concepts and theories in the development of a curriculum plan.

- Critically examines concepts and theories related to curriculum design.
- Creates a curriculum design congruent with the theory of Man-Living-Health.

Conceptual Focus:

Module I: Curriculum Development Process

Goals: To utilize the process of inquiry.

To understand the curriculum process.

Module II: Curriculum Plan

Goals: To utilize the process of inquiry.

To utilize concepts and theories in the development of a curriculum plan.

Instructional Strategies:

Faculty-student process

Student-group process

Presentation of curriculum plan

Evaluation: Evaluation is based on the achievement of the goals of the course as evidenced by:

- Performance as group leader
- Quality of curriculum plan
- Performance in presentation of curriculum plan
- Performance on final examination

■

Course Title: Teaching Nursing Practicum

Course Description: This course provides an opportunity to test the concepts and theories of Man-Living-Health, learning, decision making, and evaluation. It emphasizes the design of an original model for teaching in a baccalaureate program based on these concepts and theories. Participants are invited to test and evaluate the model through teaching in a baccalaureate program.

Goals and Indicators:

To utilize the process of inquiry.

- Uses a systematic method in approaching the leadership role of teaching nursing.

- Uses research findings to design a model for teaching nursing.
- Specifies value priorities in designing a model for teaching nursing.
- Compares various perspectives as part of decision making.
- Makes judgments based on a theoretical perspective.
- Demonstrates self-direction in testing the model for teaching nursing.
- Demonstrates accountability to self, students, and peer professionals.

To develop a structural model for teaching nursing.

- Analyzes the role of teaching nursing in institutions of higher learning.
- Synthesizes concepts and theories of Man-Living-Health, learning, decision making, and evaluation into an original model for teaching nursing.

To test the structural model in a nursing educational setting.

- Tests teaching model in a baccalaureate nursing program.
- Promotes the delivery of quality health care through teaching nursing.
- Teaches nursing from the theoretical base of Man-Living-Health.
- Promotes change in the educational system based on a theoretical perspective.
- Compares value priorities in decision making related to teaching nursing.
- Develops criteria to evaluate the effectiveness of the teaching model.

- Evaluates the effectiveness of the model for teaching nursing.

Conceptual Focus:

Module I:	Teaching Nursing Model
Goals:	To utilize the process of inquiry.
	To develop a structural model for teaching nursing.
Module II:	Responsibilities Inherent in Being a Teacher of Nursing
Goals:	To utilize the process of inquiry.
	To test the structural model in a nursing educational setting.

Instructional Strategies:

Faculty-student process

Student-student process

Teacher-student process

Student-group process

Evaluation: Evaluation is based on achievement of the goals of the course as evidenced by:

- Performance as group leader
- Quality of teaching model
- Quality of testing the teaching model
- Quality of the critique of the teaching model
- Performance in role of teacher with students
- Performance in peer review
- Performance on final examination

ADMINISTERING NURSING SERVICES
ROLE AREA: REQUIRED COURSES

Course Title: Administrative Process

Course Description: This course provides an opportunity to study concepts and theories related to administration of nursing services from the perspective of various theorists. It emphasizes the elements of the administrative process. Participants are invited to design an administrative plan from the perspective of Man-Living-Health. The plan includes philosophy, goals and indicators, conceptual framework, and an evaluation plan.

Goals and Indicators:

To utilize the process of inquiry.

- Uses a systematic method to study concepts and theories related to the administrative process.
- Uses research findings to validate administrative strategies.
- Compares various perspectives as part of decision making in the administrative process.
- Specifies value priorities in decision making related to the administrative process.
- Demonstrates self-direction in studying the administrative process.
- Demonstrates accountability to self and peer professionals.

To understand the administrative process.

- Analyzes various theories of administration.
- Critically examines the interpersonal process related to the administrative process.

To utilize concepts and theories in the development of an administrative plan.

- Critically examines concepts and theories related to the administrative process.
- Creates an administrative plan congruent with the theory of Man-Living-Health.

Conceptual Focus:
   Module I: Structure of Administrative Process
   Goals: To utilize the process of inquiry.
                To understand the administrative process.
   Module II: Administrative Plan
   Goals: To utilize the process of inquiry.
                To utilize concepts and theories in the development of an administrative plan.

Instructional Strategies:
   Faculty-student process
   Student-group process
   Presentation of administrative plan

Evaluation: Evaluation is based on the achievement of the goals of the course as evidenced by:

- Performance as group leader
- Quality of administrative plan
- Performance in presentation of administrative plan
- Performance on final examination

■

Course Title: Administering Nursing Service Practicum
Course Description: This course provides an opportunity to test the concepts and theories of Man-Living-Health, learning, decision making, and evaluation. It emphasizes the design of an original model for administering nursing services based on these concepts and theories. Participants are invited to test and evaluate the model through participating in administering nursing services in a health care agency.
Goals and Indicators:
   To utilize the process of inquiry.

- Uses a systematic method of study in approaching the leadership role of administering nursing services.
- Uses research findings to design a model for administering nursing services.
- Specifies value priorities in designing a model for administering nursing services.
- Compares various perspectives as part of decision making.
- Makes value judgments based on a theoretical perspective.
- Demonstrates self-direction in testing the model for administering nursing services.
- Demonstrates accountability to self and peer professionals.

To develop a structural model for administering nursing services.

- Analyzes health care systems.
- Synthesizes concepts and theories of Man-Living-Health, learning, decision making, and evaluation into an original model for administering nursing services.

To test the structural model in a health care setting.

- Tests administering nursing services model in a health care agency.
- Promotes the delivery of quality health care through administering nursing services.
- Administers nursing services from the theoretical base of Man-Living-Health.
- Promotes change in the health care agency based on a theoretical perspective.
- Compares value priorities in decision making related to administering nursing services.

- Develops criteria to evaluate the effectiveness of the administering nursing services model.
- Evaluates the effectiveness of the model for administering nursing services.

Conceptual Focus:

Module I: Administering Nursing Service Model

Goals: To utilize the process of inquiry.

To develop a structural model for administering nursing services.

Module II: Responsibilities Inherent in Being a Nurse Administrator

Goals: To utilize the process of inquiry.

To test the structural model in a health care setting.

Instructional Strategies:

Faculty-student process

Student-student process

Administrator-nurse process

Student-group process

Evaluation: Evaluation is based on achievement of the goals of the course as evidenced by:

- Performance as group leader
- Quality of administering nursing services model
- Quality of the critique of the administering nursing services model
- Quality of testing the administering nursing services model
- Performance in role of nurse administrator
- Performance in peer review
- Performance on final examination

Role Electives

Students may select any three of the following five courses to fulfill the role area requirements. These elective courses are three credits each and didactic.

Course Title: Nursing Leadership and Technological Resources

Course Description: This course provides an opportunity to study concepts and theories related to science and technology in leadership roles. It emphasizes the use of technological advances in nursing leadership situations. Participants are invited to consider ways of maximizing the use of technological resources for transforming nursing systems. Participants will have an opportunity to relate computer technology to nursing leadership situations.

Goals and Indicators:

To utilize the process of inquiry.

- Uses a systematic method of inquiry in examining the meaning of technology for nursing leadership.
- Uses research findings to substantiate the use of technology in specific leadership situations.
- Demonstrates self-direction in studying use of technological resources in nursing leadership.
- Delineates value priorities in use of technological resources.
- Demonstrates accountability to self and peer professionals.
- Compares various perspectives relative to the use of technology in nursing leadership situations.

To understand the relationship of sciences and technology to nursing leadership.

- Critically examines the meaning of science and technology.
- Relates science and technology to nursing leadership.

To explore the use of technological resources in nursing leadership.

- Identifies evolving technological strategies for use in nursing leadership situations.
- Synthesizes technological methodologies into a plan for transforming nursing leadership situations.

Conceptual Focus:

Module I: Science and Technology

Goals: To utilize the process of inquiry.

To understand the relationship of science and technology to nursing leadership.

Module II: Use of Technological Resources in Leadership Situations

Goals: To utilize the process of inquiry.

To explore the use of technological resources in nursing leadership.

Instructional Strategies:

Faculty-student process

Student-student process

Student-group process

Individual project related to information processing

Evaluation: Evaluation is based on achievement of the goals of the course as evidenced by:

- Performance as group leader
- Quality of project
- Performance in peer review

■

Course Title: Political Issues in Nursing Leadership

Course Description: This course provides an opportunity to study various political issues and nursing leadership. It emphasizes nursing's participation in health policy making and legal-ethical-moral responsibilities inherent in leadership roles. Participants are invited to select at least two political issues significant for nursing leadership and develop leadership strategies relative to promoting participation in the political process for the powering of nursing as an independent discipline.

Goals and Indicators:

To utilize the process of inquiry.

- Uses a systematic method of study to investigate political issues relevant to nursing leadership.
- Uses appropriate literature to substantiate positions on political issues.
- Demonstrates self-direction in relation to study of political issues.
- Delineates value priorities in relation to political issues.
- Demonstrates accountability to self and peer professionals.

To understand the relationship of health policy making to the advancement of nursing.

- Critically examines the meaning of political policy making for nursing.
- Plans strategies for nursing participation in health policy making.

To understand the legal-ethical-moral responsibilities inherent in leadership roles.

- Critically examines the various legal-ethical-moral dimensions in leadership roles.
- Identifies the responsibilities of nurse leaders in the powering of nursing through the political process.

Conceptual Focus:

Module I: Participation in Health Policy Making

Goals: To utilize the process of inquiry.

To understand the relationship of health policy making to the advancement of nursing.

Module II: Legal-Ethical-Moral Responsibilities in Nursing Leadership Roles

Goals: To utilize the process of inquiry.

To understand the legal-ethical-moral responsibilities inherent in leadership roles.

Instructional Strategies:

Faculty-student process

Student-student process

Student-group process

Group project related to political issue

Individual project related to political issue

Evaluation: Evaluation is based on achievement of the goals of the course as evidenced by:

- Performance as group leader
- Quality of group project
- Quality of individual project
- Performance in peer review

■

Course Title: Comparative Studies in Nursing Leadership

Course Description: This course provides an opportunity to study nursing leadership in different cultures. It emphasizes the examination of nursing leadership as related to powering and valuing. Participants are invited to compare and contrast the nursing educational and nursing administration frameworks of the People's Republic of China and the Soviet Union with that of the United States.

Goals and Indicators:

To utilize the process of inquiry.

- Uses a systematic method of inquiry to compare the nursing leadership structure of different cultures.
- Uses appropriate literature to substantiate a comparison of nursing leadership in different cultures.
- Demonstrates self-direction in studying the nursing leadership structure of different cultures.
- Delineates value priorities in comparing the nursing leadership structures of different cultures.
- Demonstrates accountability to self and peer professionals.

To understand the nursing leadership structure of the People's Republic of China.

- Critically examines the nursing education system of China as it relates to the value priorities of the people.
- Critically examines the administration of nursing services structure of China as it relates to the value priorities of the people.
- Compares the nursing educational system of China with that of the United States in light of power relationships.
- Compares the administration of nursing services

structure of China with that of the United States in light of power relationships.

To understand the nursing leadership structure of the Soviet Union.

- Critically examines the nursing educational system in the Soviet Union as it relates to the value priorities of the people.
- Critically examines the administration of nursing services structure in the Soviet Union as it relates to the value priorities of the people.
- Compares the nursing educational system of the Soviet Union with that of the United States in light of power relationships.
- Compares the administration of nursing services structure of the Soviet Union with that of the United States in light of power relationships.

Conceptual Focus:

Module I: Education and Administration in the People's Republic of China

Goals: To utilize the process of inquiry.

To understand the nursing leadership structure of the People's Republic of China.

Module II: Education and Administration in the Soviet Union

Goals: To utilize the process of inquiry.

To understand the nursing leadership structure of the Soviet Union.

Instructional Strategies:

Faculty-student process

Student-group process

Evaluation: Evaluation is based on achievement of the goals of the course as evidenced by:

- Performance as group leader
- Quality of one paper related to comparison of two nursing leadership systems

■

Course Title: Nursing Leadership and Health Care Systems

Course Description: This course provides an opportunity to study nursing leadership and health care systems. It emphasizes peer professional relationships in multicultural health care systems. Participants are invited to design and test change strategies relative to transforming nursing as part of a health care system.

Goals and Indicators:

To utilize the process of inquiry.

- Uses a systematic method to study nursing leadership and health care systems.
- Uses research findings to substantiate judgments relative to change strategies in health care systems.
- Demonstrates self-direction in studying nursing leadership and health care systems.
- Delineates value priorities in studying nursing leadership and health care systems.
- Compares various perspectives related to transforming nursing in multicultural health care systems.
- Demonstrates accountability to self and peer professionals.

To understand the multicultural nature of peer professional relationships in health care systems.

- Critically examines the multicultural nature of health care systems.
- Analyzes peer relationships in a multicultural system.

To test a change strategy for transforming nursing in a multicultural health care system.

- Designs a change strategy for transforming nursing in a multicultural health care system.
- Implements a change strategy for transforming nursing in a multicultural health care system.
- Evaluates the effectiveness of a change strategy for transforming nursing in a multicultural health care system.

Conceptual Focus:

Module I:	Peer Professional Relationships
Goals:	To utilize the process of inquiry.
	To understand the multicultural nature of peer professional relationships in health care systems.
Module II:	Change Strategies in a Multicultural System
Goals:	To utilize the process of inquiry.
	To test a change strategy for transforming nursing in a multicultural health care system.

Instructional Strategies:

Faculty-student process

Student-group process

Individual project related to change strategy in a health care system

Evaluation: Evaluation is based on achievement of the goals of the course as evidenced by:

- Performance as group leader
- Quality of project

■

Course Title: Nursing Leadership and Institutions of Higher Learning

Course Description: This course provides an opportunity to study nursing leadership and institutions of higher learning. It emphasizes the role of nursing leadership in promulgating nursing as an academic discipline in educational institutional systems. Participants are invited to design and test strategies relative to transforming the image of nursing in academia.

Goals and Indicators:

To utilize the process of inquiry.

- Uses a systematic method to study nursing leadership and institutions of higher learning.
- Uses research findings to substantiate judgments relative to change strategies in institutions of higher learning.
- Demonstrates self-direction in studying nursing leadership and institutions of higher learning.
- Delineates value priorities in studying nursing leadership and institutions of higher learning.
- Compares various perspectives related to transforming nursing's image in institutions of higher learning.
- Demonstrates accountability to self and peer professionals.

To understand the position of nursing among academic disciplines in institutions of higher learning.

- Critically examines the role of nursing leadership in promulgating nursing as an academic discipline in educational institutions.
- Analyzes the position of nursing among academic disciplines in institutions of higher learning.

To test a change strategy for transforming nursing's image in an institution of higher learning.

- Designs a change strategy for transforming nursing's image in an institution of higher learning.

- Implements a change strategy for transforming nursing's image in academia.
- Evaluates the effectiveness of a change strategy for transforming nursing's image in academia.

Conceptual Focus:

Module I: Academic Disciplines

Goals: To utilize the process of inquiry.

          To understand the position of nursing among academic disciplines in institutions of higher learning.

Module II: Change Strategies in Academia

Goals: To utilize the process of inquiry.

          To test a change strategy for transforming nursing's image in an institution of higher learning.

Instructional Strategies:

Faculty-student process

Student-group process

Individual project related to change strategy in academia

Evaluation: Evaluation is based on achievement of the goals of the course as evidenced by:

- Performance as group leader
- Quality of project

Sample Evaluation Plan

The evaluation plan for this proposed program leading to a master of science degree in nursing would be developed before its inception and would be consistent with the conceptual framework and philosophy of the program. A sample model is illustrated in Schema 10. The model demonstrates details related to the areas of input, output, process, supplemental, and financial, the five major elements of program evaluation.

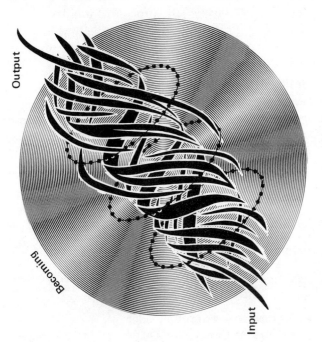

Supplemental

- What are the opinions of graduates, employees, and families

Financial

- Cost of program

Output

Becoming

Input

Input

- Initial status of students

  What are the student characteristics and level of knowledge about man—living—health?

Process

- Execution of program

  Are the courses being taught according to the curriculum plan?

Output

- Later status of students

  What have students learned after certain periods of instruction

SCHEMA 10. SAMPLE GRADUATE
NURSING PROGRAM EVALUATION MODEL

Key: Helix: openness, diversity and complexity in the learning process.

Beaded circles: levels I and II and program output relative to goals and indicators.

Concentric background: mutual and simultaneous man-environment interchange.

INPUT

Input data includes pretest scores and student characteristics. The pretest questions are general questions related to the overall program goals.

Sample Pretest Questions

1. Explain the principles of the theory of Man-Living-Health.
2. Identify three concepts of the theory of Man-Living-Health. Explain their meaning and describe a situation in nursing practice from this perspective.
3. Explain the process of concept development and theory evolution.
4. Create a proposition congruent with the theory of Man-Living-Health related to administering nursing services and from it evolve strategies for transforming.

A sample form for data collection relative to the initial status of students for the proposed master's program follows:

STUDENT CHARACTERISTICS

Circle the correct information.

Name _____ Date of birth _____

Sex: M   F   Race: Black   White   Other

Marital Status: Single   Married   Separated   Divorced

Education: B.S.N.   A.D. + B.S.N.

                        Diploma + B.S.N.   B.S.N. + Master's

                        Other Baccalaureate + B.S.N.

University where
B.S.N. received: _____

Number of years work experience after B.S.N.: _____

Type of work: Teaching

                      Administration

                      Community

                      Other

Fellowships or scholarships received: _____

Academic honors: _____

Intended role area of concentration:

                      Teaching   Administration

Millers Analogy score: _____

Graduate Record Examination score: _____

B.S.N. Quality Point average: _____

Academic reference: Positive   Neutral   Negative

Professional reference: Positive   Neutral   Negative

Preadmission interview:

                      Highly recommended

                      Recommended

                      Recommended with reservations

Student status of admission: Regular   Provisional

Pretest score: _____

OUTPUT

Output data include information collected at the end of each course, at the end of each level, and at the end of the program.

Course End Data

At the end of each course students and faculty evaluate the students' performance in light of the course goals. For example, in all courses a form such as the following for Nursing Science: Man-Living-Health would be used to gather data. Students and faculty would complete the form.

COURSE END EVALUATION
NURSING SCIENCE: MAN-LIVING-HEALTH

Student name:

Goals and Indicators:

To utilize the process of inquiry.

	Unable to Rate	Outstanding	Good	Satisfactory	Marginally Satisfactory	Marginally Unsatisfactory	Unsatisfactory
• Examines systematically the elements of the theory of Man-Living-Health.							
• Uses literature to support convictions.							
• Delineates value priorities in qualifying convictions.							
• Demonstrates self-direction in studying Man-Living-Health.							

To understand the assumptions underpinning the theory of Man-Living-Health.

- Examines the concepts synthesized in each assumption.
- Compares the meaning of each assumption.
- Synthesizes the meaning of the assumptions as a basis for nursing practice.

To comprehend the theory of Man-Living-Health.

- Examines the principles, concepts, and theoretical structures of Man-Living-Health.
- Relates each principle to the basic assumptions of the theory.
- Relates the theoretical structures to nursing practice.

At the end of each course, students would also complete a form such as the following for Nursing Science: Man-Living-Health relative to the conduct of the course.

STUDENT COURSE END EVALUATION
NURSING SCIENCE: MAN-LIVING-HEALTH

Please mark an "x" in the appropriate box.

1. How clear was the presentation of material in Nursing Science: Man-Living-Health?

   Clear ☐ ☐ ☐ ☐ Unclear

2. How would you rate this course as compared to others?

   Difficult ☐ ☐ ☐ ☐ Easy

3. How helpful were the readings in helping you to learn?

   Helpful ☐ ☐ ☐ ☐ Not helpful

4. How much difficulty did you have in following the concepts taught in the course?

   Little ☐ ☐ ☐ ☐ Much

5. How would you rate the amount of work that was required in this course?

   Much ☐ ☐ ☐ ☐ Little

6. How clear were the expectations of the course?

   Clear ☐ ☐ ☐ ☐ Unclear

7. How free were you to express your own ideas in this course?

   Free ☐ ☐ ☐ ☐ Not free

8. Do you feel you were given enough opportunity to clarify your thoughts?

   Yes ☐ No ☐

9. How helpful was didactic presentation to your learning?

   Helpful ☐ ☐ ☐ ☐ Not helpful

10. How helpful to your learning were the two required papers?

Helpful ☐   ☐   ☐   ☐   Not helpful

Final examinations are given in all required courses except for Nursing Research II in this proposed graduate nursing program. A sample test question for the course Nursing Science: Man-Living-Health in the proposed program follows:

• Explain the meaning of one theoretical structure from the theory of Man-Living-Health as it relates to the practice of nursing with families.

Level End Data

At the end of each level the faculty members teaching at the level would evaluate each student's performance. Each faculty member, individually, would evaluate each student, and then all faculty members from that particular level would meet and discuss their individual decisions relative to each indicator for each student. The faculty members' collective rating of a student is the student's final rating on an indicator at a particular level.

Sample Level I and Level II evaluation forms for this proposed master's curriculum follow:

LEVEL I INDICATORS

(evaluation after 24 credits)

	Unable to Rate	Outstanding	Good	Satisfactory	Marginally Satisfactory	Marginally Unsatisfactory	Unsatisfactory
Program Goal I:							
To practice in a leadership role nursing based on the theory of Man-Living-Health.							
• Comprehends concepts related to Man-Living-Health.							
• Illuminates patterns of relating with families.							
• Demonstrates self-direction.							
• Demonstrates accountability to families.							
• Initiates collaborative relationship with families and peer professionals.							

Program Goal II:

To practice a leadership role of teaching nursing or administering nursing services from the theoretical base of Man-Living-Health.							
• Identifies quality health care from the perspective of Man-Living-Health.							
• Identifies change strategies related to theoretical perspectives.							
• Incorporates principles of teaching or administration with the theory of Man-Living-Health.							
• Compares value priorities relative to nursing issues.							
• Demonstrates accountability to self and peer professionals.							

(continued)

161

Program Goal III:

To utilize the process of inquiry.

	Unable to Rate	Outstanding	Good	Satisfactory	Marginally Satisfactory	Marginally Unsatisfactory	Unsatisfactory
• Uses a systematic method to study concepts of Man-Living-Health.							
• Uses literature to support conclusions.							
• Comprehends the elements of the theory of Man-Living-Health.							
• Examines various perspectives related to nursing issues.							

162

• Identifies judgments as based on theoretical foundations.						
• Delineates value priorities in qualifying convictions.						
Program Goal IV:						
To contribute to theory evolution in nursing.						
• Develops concepts from the perspective of Man-Living-Health relevant for nursing.						
• Compares extant nursing theories.						

LEVEL II INDICATORS

(evaluation after 48 credits)

Program Goal I:

To practice in a leadership role nursing based on the theory of Man-Living-Health.

	Unable to Rate	Outstanding	Good	Satisfactory	Marginally Satisfactory	Marginally Unsatisfactory	Unsatisfactory
• Understands concepts related to Man-Living-Health.							
• Guides families in choosing possibilities in their changing health process.							
• Demonstrates self-direction.							

• Demonstrates accountability to families.						
• Initiates collaborative relationships with families and peer professionals.						
Program Goal II:						
To practice a leadership role of teaching nursing or administering nursing services from the theoretical base of Man-Living-Health						
• Promotes the delivery of quality health care through teaching nursing or administering nursing services.						
• Promotes change in social systems based on the theoretical perspective of Man-Living-Health.						

(continued)

165

	Unable to Rate	Outstanding	Good	Satisfactory	Marginally Satisfactory	Marginally Unsatisfactory	Unsatisfactory
• Teaches nursing or administers nursing services from the theoretical base of Man-Living-Health.							
• Compares value priorities in decision making.							
• Demonstrates accountability to self and peer professionals.							
Program Goal III:							
To utilize the process of inquiry.							
• Uses a systematic method of study in nursing.							

• Uses research findings to enhance decision making.									
• Tests the theory of Man-Living-Health.									
• Compares various perspectives as part of decision making.									
• Makes judgments based on a theoretical perspective.									
• Specifies value priorities in decision making.									
Program Goal IV:									
To contribute to theory evolution in nursing.									
• Develops concepts from the perspective of Man-Living-Health relevant for nursing.									
• Validates concepts for their applicability to the theory of Man-Living-Health.									

A similar form and procedure would be used for program end evaluation of students.

PROCESS

Process data are collected relative to program execution for the proposed program. A few questions shown on the following sample form, used for the course Nursing Science: Man-Living-Health, might be used by the evaluator for class visitation.

The evaluator would also inspect course materials such as printed materials, student papers, and projects to determine if these, in fact, reflect the course goals.

SUPPLEMENTAL

Supplemental data would be collected from faculty, students, families, program graduates, and supervisors. Faculty members and students would be interviewed by the evaluator of the program relative to their opinions about the program. Sample interview questions are as follows:

Faculty and Students
1. What do you see as the major strengths of the program?
2. What do you see as the major limitations of the program?
3. Describe how you would recreate the program to strengthen it.

Families
Families would be interviewed to determine their opinions of the program as experienced through the students who visited them. Families might be asked questions such as the following:

1. Did you understand why the graduate nursing student met with you?

CLASS VISITATION
NURSING SCIENCE: MAN-LIVING-HEALTH

	Yes	No	Other comments
1. The students express their ideas during class.			
2. Students are given the opportunity to ask questions.			
3. Student-group process is a teaching method in this course.			
4. The main method of presentation is discussion.			
5. Printed materials are distributed to the class.			
6. The principles and concepts of the theory of Man-Living-Health are discussed.			
7. Assumptions about man and health are discussed.			
8. Students can state the course goals.			
9. Students systematically present concepts.			

2. Did you find the student's contact with your family beneficial?

3. Describe in what way you would like to see the visits changed.

Program Graduates

Program graduates would be surveyed at six months, one year, and five years after graduation to ascertain their opinions of their educational experience in light of the program goals.

A few sample questions in a six-month evaluation survey form for this proposed master's program follows:

1. How would you rate your satisfaction with the quality of instruction in your master's program? (circle one)

   extremely satisfactory   not satisfactory
   moderately satisfactory   unable to evaluate

2. How worthwhile was the program in light of your job responsibilities? (circle one)

   extremely worthwhile   not worthwhile
   moderately worthwhile   unable to evaluate

3. How satisfactory was the overall structure of the program? (circle one)

   extremely satisfactory   not satisfactory
   moderately satisfactory   unable to evaluate

Supervisors

Immediate supervisors of the graduates would be surveyed at six months and one year after graduation to ascertain the performance level of the graduates in light of the program goals. A few sample questions on a six-month supervisor survey form for this proposed masters program follows:

1. How would you rate the *overall* performance of the graduate? (circle one)

   very poor   good

   poor   very good

   satisfactory   oustanding

           unable to evaluate

2. In the graduate's work situation, how important is it that she demonstrates the ability to provide services to families? (circle one)

   important   not important

3. If it is important that the graduate have ability to provide families, how would you rate the graduate's performance in this area? (circle one)

   very poor   good

   poor   very good

   satisfactory   outstanding

           unable to evaluate

4. In the graduate's work situation, how important is it that she have ability to initiate change? (circle one)

   important   not important

5. If it is important that the graduate have the ability to initiate change, how would you rate the graduate's performance in this area?

   very poor   good

   poor   very good

   satisfactory   outstanding

           unable to evaluate

FINANCIAL

All costs for the proposed program would be categorized into direct or indirect, basic or additional, and recurring or nonrecurring costs.

The data from all the above categories—input, output, process, supplemental, and financial—would be ordered and interpreted in light of the program philosophy and goals and the evaluation model. The results would be used as a basis for decision making about the proposed program.

The sample curriculum plan for a program leading to a master of science in nursing degree details the theory of Man-Living-Health as the theoretical base of a graduate nursing program. It is through the nursing education programs that are grounded in theory that nursing's body of knowledge is disseminated to those who practice, teach, and research. Quality and scholarliness in these programs is essential to the advancement of nursing.

The theory of nursing rooted in the human sciences, presented in this book, provides a foundation from which new questions can be raised about the phenomenon of nursing. The emergence of nursing as a science and an art is through creative conceptualization in research, practice, and education. Nursing is unfolding in simultaneous and mutual interchange with the world transcending with greater diversity and complexity. Nursing is all at once what it was, is, and will become, growing ever more explicit but always with the mystery of the not-yet.

Epilogue

Mary Jane Smith, Ph.D., R.N.

This work, *Man-Living-Health: A Theory of Nursing*, presents a call to nurses who wish to cultivate the growing edge of the field of nursing. To cultivate can be likened to tilling the soil, which is an uncovering of that which lies hidden. The digging and probing in tilling loosens and enlivens the ground while nourishing growth and fruitfulness. The cultivating of a paradigm of nursing is a personal commitment related to one's belief system or worldview. The worldview is the paradigm that gives meaning to what one does in research, practice, and teaching. One's worldview guides the digging and probing of scientific endeavors by structuring the process of questioning and answering.

To participate in cultivating at the growing edge of nursing as a researcher, practitioner, or teacher, where knowledge and values are shifting and changing, is a risky endeavor rich with opportunities to advance nursing science. Not everyone will choose to venture out into the growing edge, where creative conceptualization, a tolerance for uncertainty, and watchful diligence are requisite.

The first requisite, creative conceptualization, is the imaginative leaping that leads one to the growing edge of the endeavors of science. This imaginative leap occurs through the process of dwelling with an idea and synthesizing knowledge in a different way. The different way includes a change in perspective arrived at through being with the tacit presence of an idea over time that flows as a mountain fog in and out of doubt. Flowing in and out of the fog of doubt is essential to conceptualizing the questions basic to gathering evidence upon which to ground nursing science.

Another requisite, a tolerance for uncertainty, is the living with ambiguity that is inherent in dwelling with the doubt spawned by differences. Bronowski states "all knowledge, all information between human beings can only be exchanged within a play of tolerance."[1] Since knowledge is a human construction, it is confined to the boundary of one's worldview. A tolerance for uncertainty is not the acceptance of bewildering logic or obscurity but, rather, patience with ambiguity leading to coherence. The seeking of coherence is a process requiring a patient gentleness with self in conceptualizing questions basic to inquiry. Patient gentleness refers to an unhurried and yet responsible way of cultivating the growing edge and requires persevering over a long period of time. Nurturing a paradigm over time calls for the third requisite: untiring, watchful diligence in which self-monitoring and discipline nourish the digging, probing, and doubting in the conceptualization of questions. Watchful diligence is an investment of personal energy reflecting one's values and commitment to contribute to nursing science at the growing edge.

It is through the processes of creative conceptualization, a tolerance for ambiguity, and watchful diligence that the growing edge of the field of nursing will be cultivated. This cultivation by researchers, practitioners, and teachers will yield empirical evidence to ground nursing science. *Man-Living-Health: A Theory of Nursing* at the growing edge. Some will risk the journey to

---

[1] Jacob Bronowski, *The Ascent of Man* (Boston: Little, Brown and Company, 1973), p. 365.

the growing edge while others will choose to remain at the center or mainstay of the field of nursing.

The hope for the future of nursing rests with those who choose to cultivate the growing edge, which is the interface of what is and what is not-yet. The cultivating takes place in the context of a community of scholars both within and against the community. A paradigm shift is both away from the center or mainstay and yet toward unity within it. Cultivating the growing edge, then, is a complex, enlivening enterprise essential to the flowering of nursing science.

Glossary

All at once Mutually simultaneous

Coexistence Living with predessors, contemporaries, and successors all at once

Coconstitution Man's active participation in creating meaning with others and the world

Concept Idea; one's conceptualization of a precept

Cocreate Initiate anew with another; coconstitute

Cotranscending Going beyond the actual in interrelationship with others

Entropy Process of becoming more homogeneous; the opposite of negentropy

Existentialism A philosophy of choosing being and becoming

Facticity What one is born to; the givens at birth

Historicity One's becoming over time

Imaging Symbolizing or picturing

Intentionality Man's nature of knowing and being present to the world

Intersubjectivity Subject-to-subject relationship involving true presence

Languaging Sharing valued images through symbols of words, gesture, gaze, touch, and posture

Living unity An experiencing subject who is more than and different from sum of parts

Meta metaperspective One's view of the other's view of the view

Metaperspective One's view of the other's view

Negentropy Process of evolving toward greater complexity

Not-yet Possibilities to be unfolded

Originating Springing from; emerging

Pattern A configuration of man-environment interrelationship

Patterns of relating An individual's way of being recognized

Paradigm A way of viewing a particular field of study

Paradox Unity of apparent opposites

Paradoxical Having an apparently contradictory nature

Perspectival view One's single-sided view of a phenomenon

Phenomenology The study of phenomena as they unfold

Possibles The imaginables toward which one reaches

Powering Struggling with the tension of pushing-resisting

Prereflective choosing Tacitly making a decision without explicit consideration

Principle A professed rule of action

Project Man's creations, including self

Reflective choosing Explicitly considering options in decision making

Rhythmical Cadent; ordered

Situated freedom Freedom to choose from options in each situation

Subjectivity A wholistic phenomenon referring to man

Synergistic Mutually and simultaneously enhancing

Tenet A basic belief

Theoretical structure A statement interrelating concepts in a way that can be verified

Transcending Going beyond; exceeding

Transforming Changing change

True presence Genuine attentiveness to the other

Valuing Choosing to confirm a cherished belief

Wholeness More than and different from the sum of
  parts.

Bibliography

Abbott, Edwin A. *Flatland.* New York: Dover Publications, 1952.

Adler, Charles S., Gene Stanford, and Sheila Morrissey, eds. *We Are But A Moment's Sunlight.* New York: Simon & Schuster, 1976.

Alinsky, Saul D. *Reveille for Radicals.* New York: Random House, 1969.

Alinsky, Saul D. *Rules for Radicals.* New York: Random House, 1972.

Anderson, Robert T. *Anthropology: A Perspective on Man.* Belmont, California: Wadsworth, 1972.

Ballard, Edward G. *Man and Technology.* Atlantic Highlands, New Jersey: Humanities Press, 1978.

Bandler, Richard, and John Grinder. *The Structure of Magic I.* Palo Alto, California: Science and Behavior Books, 1975.

Bandler, Richard, and John Grinder. *Patterns of the Hypnotic Techniques of Milton H. Erickson.* Vol. I. Cupertino, California: Meta Publications, 1975.

Bannon, John F. *The Philosophy of Merleau-Ponty.* New York: Harcourt, Brace and World, 1967.

Barnett, Lincoln. *The Universe and Dr. Einstein.* New York: Bantam Books, 1948.

Barrett, William. *What is Existentialism?* New York: Grove Press, 1965.

Belgium, D. R., ed. *Religion and Medicine: Essays of Meaning, Valuing and Health.* Ames, Iowa: Iowa State University Press, 1967.

Bentov, Itzhak. *Stalking the Wild Pendulum.* New York: E. P. Dutton, 1977.

Berger, Peter L., and Thomas Luckmann. *The Social Construction of Reality.* New York: Doubleday, 1966.

Besant, Annie. *Thought Power: Its Control and Culture.* Wheaton, Illinois: Theosophical Publishing House, 1903.

Bok, Sissela. *Lying: Moral Choice in Public and Private Life.* New York: Pantheon Books, 1978.

Bolen, Jean Shinoda. *The Tao of Psychology: Synchronicity and the Self.* San Francisco: Harper & Row, 1979.

Born, Max. *Einstein's Theory of Relativity.* Rev. ed. New York: Dover Publications, 1962.

Bruner, Jerome S. *The Process of Education.* New York: Random House, 1960.

Bruteau, Beatrice. *The Psychic Grid.* Wheaton, Illinois: Theosophical Publishing House, 1979.

Buber, Martin. *The Knowledge of Man.* Edited by Maurice Friedman. New York: Harper & Row, 1965.

Buber, Martin. *I and Thou.* New York: Charles Scribner's Sons, 1970.

Buytendyk, F. J. J. *Prolegomena to an Anthropological Physiology.* Atlantic Highlands, New Jersey: Humanities Press, 1974.

Calder, Nigel. *Einstein's Universe.* New York: The Viking Press, 1979.

Campbell, Joseph. *The Hero with a Thousand Faces.* Princeton, New Jersey: Princeton University Press, 1959.

Camus, Albert. *The Stranger.* New York: Random House, 1946.

Capra, Fritjof. *The Tao of Physics.* New York: Bantam Books, 1976.

Carroll, Lewis. *The Annotated Alice: Alice's Adventures in Wonderland and Through the Looking Glass.* Cleveland and New York: World Publishing Company, 1960.

Castaneda, Carlos. *Journey to Ixtlan: The Lessons of Don Juan.* New York: Simon & Schuster, 1972.

Castaneda, Carlos. *Tales of Power.* New York: Simon & Schuster, 1974.

Castaneda, Carlos. *The Second Ring of Power.* New York: Simon & Schuster, 1977.

Colaizzi, Paul F. *Technology and Dwelling: The Secrets of Life and Death,* 1978.

Collingwood, R. D. *The Idea of History.* New York: Oxford University Press, 1956.

Darwin, Charles. *Origin of Species.* New York: Hill and Wang, 1979.

de Beauvoir, Simone. *The Ethics of Ambiguity.* Secaucus, New Jersey: Citadel Press, 1948.

de Beauvoir, Simone. *A Very Easy Death.* New York: Warner Books, 1977.

de Bono, Edward. *New Think.* New York: The Hearst Corporation, 1967.

de Chardin, Teilhard. *The Phenomenon of Man.* New York: Harper & Row, 1965.

de Chardin, Teilhard. *On Love and Suffering.* New York: Paulist Press, 1966.

Dilthey, Wilhelm. *Pattern and Meaning in History.* New York: Harper & Row, 1961.

Dubin, Robert. *Theory Building.* New York: The Free Press, 1969.

Dubos, René. *Man Adapting.* New Haven, Connecticut: Yale University Press, 1970.

Einstein, Albert. *The Meaning of Relativity.* Princeton, New Jersey: Princeton University Press, 1946.

Ellis, Rosemary. "Fallabilities, Fragments and Frames: Contemplations on 25 years of Research in Medical-Surgical Nursing." *Nursing Research* 26 (3): 181, May-June 1977.

Englehardt, H. Tristram Jr., and Daniel Callahan, eds. *Knowledge, Value and Belief.* Vol. II. New York: The Hastings Center, Institute of Society, Ethics and The Life Sciences, 1977.

Evans-Wenty, W. Y. The *Tibetan Book of the Dead.* London: Oxford University Press, 1978.

Feifel, Herman, ed. *The Meaning of Death.* New York: McGraw-Hill, 1965.

Ferguson, Marilyn, *The Aquarian Conspiracy: Personal and Social Transformation in the 1980's.* Los Angeles: J. P. Tarcher, 1980.

Fischer, Constance T., and Stanley L. Brodsky, eds. *Client Participation in Human Services: The Prometheus Principle.* New Brunswick, New Jersey: Transaction, 1978.

Fisher, Alden L. *The Essential Writings of Merleau-Ponty.* New York: Harcourt, Brace and World, 1969.

Fletcher, Joseph. *Situation Ethics.* Philadelphia: The Westminster Press, 1975.

Frankl, Viktor E. *The Doctor and the Soul.* New York: Alfred A. Knopf, 1960.

Frankl, Viktor E. *The Will to Meaning.* New York: New American Library, 1969.

Frankl, Viktor E. *Man's Search for Meaning.* New York: Simon & Schuster, 1972.

Frazier, Claude A. *Faith Healing: Finger of God? or*

Scientific Curiosity? New York: Thomas Nelson, 1974.

Fromm, Erich. *The Art of Loving.* New York: Harper & Row, 1963.

Fromm, Erich. *The Revolution of Hope.* New York: Harper & Row, 1968.

Gary, William, Fredrick J. Duhl, and Nicholas D. Rizzo, eds. *General Systems Theory and Psychiatry.* Boston: Little, Brown & Company, 1969.

Gaylin, Willard. *Feelings.* New York: Harper & Row, 1979.

Ghiselin, Brewster, ed. *The Creative Process.* Berkeley, California: University of California Press, 1952.

Giorgi, Amedeo. *Psychology as a Human Science.* New York: Harper & Row, 1970.

Giorgi, Amedeo, Richard Knowles, and David L. Smith, eds. *Phenomenological Psychology.* Vol. III. Pittsburgh: Duquesne University Press, 1979.

Goffman, Erving. *The Presentation of Self in Everyday Life.* New York: Doubleday Anchor Books, 1959.

Goffman, Erving. *Asylums.* New York: Doubleday Anchor Books, 1961.

Goffman, Erving. *Interactional Ritual: Essays on Face-to-Face Behavior.* Garden City, New York: Doubleday Anchor Books, 1967.

Goffman, Erving. *Frame Analysis.* New York: Harper & Row, 1974.

Gordon, David. *Therapeutic Metaphors.* Cupertino, California: Meta Publications, 1978.

Greene, Maxine. *Landscapes of Learning.* New York: Teachers College Press, 1978.

Grinder, John, and Richard Bandler. *The Structure of Magic II.* Palo Alto, California: Science and Behavior Books, 1976.

Habermas, Jurgen. *Knowledge and Human Interests.* Boston: Beacon Press, 1968.

Hageman, Louise. *In the Midst of Winter.* Denville, New Jersey: Dimension Books, 1977.

Hall, Edward T. *Beyond Culture.* Garden City, New York: Doubleday Anchor Books, 1976.

Hall, Brian P. *The Development of Consciousness: A Confluent Theory of Values.* New York: Paulist Press, 1976.

Heidegger, Martin. *On Time and Being.* New York: Harper & Row, 1972.

Heidegger, Martin. *Being and Time.* New York: Harper & Row, 1962.

Hempel, Carl G. *Philosophy of Natural Science.* Engelwood Cliffs, New Jersey: Prentice-Hall, 1966.

Henderson, Virginia. "The Nature of Nursing." *American Journal of Nursing* 64 (8), August 1964, pp 62–68.

Jourard, Sidney M. *The Transparent Self.* New York: D. Van Nostrand, 1971.

Kaplan, Abraham. *The New World of Philosophy.* New York: Random House, 1961.

Kaplan, Abraham. *The Conduct of Inquiry: Methodology for Behavioral Sciences.* Scranton, Pennsylvania: Chandler Publishing Company, 1964.

Keen, Sam. *Apology for Wonder.* New York: Harper & Row, 1960.

Keen, Sam. *Gabriel Marcel.* Richmond, Virginia: John Knox Press, 1967.

Keen, Sam. *To A Dancing God.* New York: Harper & Row, 1970.

Keleman, Stanley. *Living Your Dying.* New York: Random House, 1975.

Kempler, Walter. *Principles of Gestalt Family Therapy.* Oslo, Norway: A.s Joh. Nordahls, Trykkeri, 1974.

Kesey, Ken. *One Flew Over the Cuckoo's Nest.* New York: The Viking Press, 1962.

King, Imogene M. *Toward a Theory for Nursing: General Concepts of Human Behavior.* New York: John Wiley & Sons, 1971.

Kockelmans, Joseph J., ed. *Phenomenology.* New York: Doubleday, 1967.

Koestler, Arthur. *Janus: A Summing Up.* New York: Vintage Books, 1974.

Kraft, William F. *A Psychology of Nothingness.* Philadelphia: Westminster Press, 1974.

Kuhn, Thomas S. *The Structure of Scientific Revolutions.* Chicago: University of Chicago Press, 1970.

Kuhns, William. *Environmental Man.* New York: Harper & Row, 1969.

Kurtz, Paul. *Exhuberance: A Philosophy of Happiness.* Buffalo: Prometheus Books, 1977.

Laing, R. D. *The Divided Self.* Baltimore, Maryland: Pelican Books, 1970.

Laing, R. D. *The Politics of Experience.* New York: Ballantine Books, 1970.

Laing, R. D. *The Politics of the Family.* New York: Random House, 1972.

Laing, R. D., H. Phillipson, and A. R. Lee. *Interpersonal Perception: A Theory and A Method of Research.* New York: Harper & Row, 1966.

Lamont, Corliss. *The Philosophy of Humanism.* New York: Frederick Ungar, 1977.

Langer, Susanne K. *Philosophy in a New Key.* Cambridge, Massachusetts: Harvard University Press, 1976.

Lasswell, Harold. *Power and Personality.* New York: W. W. Norton, 1976.

Lasswell, Harold. *Politics: Who Gets What, When, How.* New York: The World Publishing Company, 1958.

Laudan, Larry. *Progress and Its Problems.* Berkeley, California: University of California Press, 1978.

Leininger, Madeleine, ed., *Transcultural Nursing Care of Infants and Children.* Salt Lake City, Utah: University of Utah College and Nursing, 1977.

Leininger, Madeleine. *Transcultural Nursing: Concepts, Theories and Practices.* New York: John Wiley & Sons, 1978.

Leonard, George. *The Transformation.* New York: Dell, 1972.

Leonard George. *The Silent Pulse.* New York: E. P. Dutton, 1978.

LeShan, Lawrence. *You Can Fight For Your Life.* New York: M. Evans and Company, 1977.

Lieber, Lillian R., and Hugh Gray Lieber. *The Einstein Theory of Relativity.* New York: Rinehart & Company, 1936.

Luijpen, William A. *Existential Phenomenology.* New York: Humanities Press, 1960.

McClelland, D. C. *Power: The Inner Experience.* New York: Irvington Publishers, 1975.

McLuhan, Marshall, and Quenton Fiore. *The Medium is the Massage.* New York: Bantam Books, 1967.

Macquarrie, John. *Martin Heidegger.* Richmond, Virginia: John Knox Press, 1968.

Mann, Felix. *Acupuncture.* New York: Random House, 1972.

Marcel, Gabriel. *The Philosophy of Existentialism.* Secaucus, New Jersey: The Citadel Press, 1956.

Marcel, Gabriel. *Creative Fidelity.* New York: The Noonday Press, 1964.

Marcel, Gabriel. *Mystery of Being: Reflection and Mystery.* Vol. I. South Bend, Indiana: Gateway Editions, 1978.

Maslow, Abraham H. *Toward a Psychology of Being.* Princeton, New Jersey: D. Van Nostrand, 1968.

Maslow, Abraham H., ed. *New Knowledge in Human Values.* Chicago: Henry Regnery, 1971.

Maslow, Abraham H. *The Farther Reaches of Human Nature.* New York: The Viking Press, 1973.

Mason, Herbert. *Gilgamesh.* New York: New American Library, with Houghton Mifflin Company, 1970.

May, Rollo. *Man's Search for Himself.* New York: W. W. Norton, 1967.

May, Rollo. *Power and Innocence: A Search for the Sources of Violence.* New York: W. W. Norton, 1972.

May, Rollo. *The Courage to Create.* Toronto, Ontario, Canada: George J. McLeod, 1975.

Mayeroff, Milton. *On Caring.* New York: Harper & Row, 1971.

Mendelsohn, Robert S. *Confessions of a Medical Heretic.* Chicago: Contemporary Books, 1979.

Merleau-Ponty, Maurice. *The Structure of Behavior.* Boston: Beacon Press, 1963.

Merleau-Ponty, Maurice. *The Prose of the World.* Evanston, Illinois: Northwestern University Press, 1973.

Merleau-Ponty, Maurice, translated by Colin Smith. *Phenomenology of Perception.* New York: Humanities Press, 1974.

Montagu, Ashley. *Touching.* New York: Harper & Row, 1972.

Montagu, Ashley, and Floyd Matson. *The Human Connection.* New York: McGraw-Hill, 1979.

Moustakas, Clark E. *Loneliness.* Englewood Cliffs, New Jersey: Prentice-Hall, 1961.

Moustakas, Clark E. *Loneliness and Love.* Englewood Cliffs, New Jersey: Prentice-Hall, 1972.

Moustakas, Clark E. *The Self.* New York: Harper & Row, 1974.

Moustakas, Clark E. *The Touch of Loneliness.* Englewood Cliffs, New Jersey: Prentice-Hall, 1975.

Moustakas, Clark E. *Creative Life.* New York: Van Nostrand Reinhold, 1977.

Natanson, Maurice, ed. *The Problem of Social Reality.* Collected Papers, Vol. I. The Hague: Martinus Nijhoff, 1967.

Newman, Margaret. *Theory Development in Nursing.* Philadelphia: F. A. Davis, 1979.

Nierenberg, Gerald I., and Henry Calero. *Meta-Talk: The Guide to Hidden Meanings in Conversation.* New York: Simon & Schuster, 1973.

Nietzsche, Friedrich. *Thus Spoke Zarathustra.* New York: The Viking Press, 1973.

Nietzsche, Friedrich. *The Will to Power.* Translated by Walter Kaufmann. New York: Vintage Books, 1968.

Nightingale, Florence. *Notes on Nursing: What It Is and What It Is Not.* Philadelphia: J. P. Lippincott, 1946. Facsimile of the First Edition printed in London, 1859.

Ogilvy, James. *Many Dimensional Man.* New York: Harper & Row, 1977.

Ornstein, Robert E. *On the Experience of Time.* New York: Penguin Books, 1969.

Ornstein, Robert E. *The Psychology of Consciousness.* San Francisco: W. H. Freeman, 1972.

Parse, Rosemarie R. *Nursing Fundamentals.* Flushing, New York: Medical Examination Publishing, 1974.

Paterson, Josephine, and Loretta T. Zderad, *Humanistic Nursing.* New York: John Wiley & Sons, 1976.

Perkins, Robert L. *Søren Kierkegaard.* Atlanta: John Knox Press, 1976.

Perls, Frederick S. *Gestalt Therapy Verbatim.* Lafayette, California: Real People Press, 1969.

Peter, Laurence J., and Raymond Hull. *The Peter Principle.* New York: Bantam Books, 1970.

Phillips, D. C. *Holistic Thought in Social Science*. Stanford, California: Stanford University Press, 1976.

Pirsig. Robert M. *Zen and the Art of Motorcycle Maintenance*. New York: Bantam Books, 1980.

Polanyi, Michael. *Personal Knowledge*. Chicago: University of Chicago Press, 1958.

Polanyi, Michael. *The Study of Man*. Chicago: University of Chicago Press, 1959.

Polanyi, Michael. *The Tacit Dimension*. Garden City, New York: Doubleday Anchor Books, 1966.

Polanyi, Michael. *Knowing and Being*. Chicago: University of Chicago Press, 1969.

Popper, Sir Karl. *The Logic of Scientific Discovery*. New York: Harper & Row, 1959.

Prather, Hugh. *I Touch the Earth, The Earth Touches Me*. Garden City, New York: Doubleday, 1972.

Prather, Hugh. *Notes on Love and Courage*. Garden City, New York: Doubleday, 1977.

Prather, Hugh. *Notes to Myself*. Moab, Utah: Real People Press, 1970.

Raths, Louis, E., Merrill Harmin, and Sidney B. Simon. *Values and Teaching: Working with Values in the Classroom*. Columbus, Ohio: Charles E. Merrill, 1978.

Reynolds, Paul Davidson. *A Primer in Theory Construction*. Indianapolis: Bobbs-Merrill, 1975.

Riehl, Joan P., and Callista Roy, *Conceptual Models for Nursing Practice*. New York: Appleton-Century-Crofts, 1980.

Rilke, Rainer Maria. *The Notebooks of Malte Lawrids Brigge*. New York: W. W. Norton, 1964.

Rogers, Carl E., and Barry Stevens. *Person to Person: The Problem of Being Human*. New York: Pocket Books, 1971.

Rogers, Martha E. *Educational Revolution in Nursing.* New York: Macmillan, 1961.

Rogers, Martha E. An *Introduction to the Theoretical Basis of Nursing.* Philadelphia: F. A. Davis, 1970.

Rosenthal, Ted. *How Could I Not Be Among You.* New York: George Braziller, 1973.

Sallis, John. *Phenomenology and the Return to Beginnings.* New York: Humanities Press, 1973.

Sapir, Edward. *Culture, Language and Personality.* Berkeley and Los Angeles: University of California Press, 1966.

Sartre, Jean-Paul. *Search for a Method.* New York: Alfred A. Knopf, 1963.

Sartre, Jean-Paul. *Nausea.* New York: New Dimensions, 1964.

Sartre, Jean-Paul. *Being and Nothingness.* New York: Washington Square Press, 1966.

Schumacher, E. F. *Small is Beautiful.* New York: Harper & Row, 1973.

Schutz, Alfred. *On Phenomenology and Social Relations.* Chicago: University of Chicago Press, 1975.

Schutz, William C. *Joy.* New York: Grove Press, 1967.

Selye, Hans. *The Stress of Life.* New York: McGraw-Hill, 1950.

Shostrom, Everett L. *Man the Manipulator.* New York: Bantam Books, 1968.

Smith, R. G. *Martin Buber.* Atlanta: John Knox Press, 1975.

Sobel, David S., ed. *Ways of Health: Holistic Approaches to Ancient and Contemporary Medicine.* New York: Harcourt Brace Jovanovich, 1979.

Sontag, Susan. *Illness as Metaphor.* New York: Vintage Books, 1979.

Spiegelberg, Herbert. *The Phenomenological Movement.* Vols. I and II. The Hague, Netherlands: Martinus Nijhoff, 1976.

Stevens, Wallace. *The Necessary Angel*. New York: Random House, 1942.

Strasser, Stephan. *Phenomenology and the Human Sciences*. Pittsburgh: Duquesne University Press, 1963.

Strasser, Stephan. *The Idea of Dialogal Phenomenology*. Pittsburgh: Duquesne University Press, 1969.

Straus, Erwin W., ed. *Language and Language Disturbances*. New York: Humanities Press, 1974.

Szasz, Thomas S. *The Myth of Mental Illness*. Rev. ed. New York: Harper & Row, 1974.

Tillich, Paul. *The Courage to Be*. New Haven: Yale University Press, 1952.

Tillich, Paul. *Love, Power, and Justice*. New York: Oxford University Press, 1954.

Tillich, Paul. *The New Being*. New York: Charles Scribner's Sons, 1955.

Tillich, Paul. *The New Eternal Now*. New York: Charles Scribner's Sons, 1963.

Toben, Bob. *Space-Time and Beyond*. New York: E. P. Dutton, 1975.

Toffler, Alvin. *Future Shock*. New York: Random House, 1970.

Toffler, Alvin, ed. *Learning for Tomorrow: The Role of the Future in Education*. New York: Random House, 1974.

Toumlin, Stephen. *The Philosophy of Science*. New York: Harper & Row, 1960.

Tournier, Paul. *The Meaning of Persons*. New York: Harper & Row, 1973.

Towers, Bernard. *Teilhard de Chardin*. Atlanta: John Knox Press, 1975.

Toynbee, Arnold. *Mankind and Mother Earth*. New York: Oxford University Press, 1976.

van den Berg, J. H. *The Psychology of the Sick Bed*. Pittsburgh: Duquesne University Press, 1966.

van den Berg, J. H. *Things: Four Metabletic Reflections.* Pittsburgh: Duquesne University Press, 1970.

van den Berg, J. H. "Phenomenology and Metabletics." *Humanitas* 7 (3). Pittsburgh: Duquesne University Press, 1973.

van Kaam, Adrian. *The Art of Existential Counseling.* Wilkes-Barre, Pennsylvania: Dimension Books, 1966.

van Kaam, Adrian. *Existential Foundations of Psychology.* New York: Doubleday, 1969.

van Kaam, Adrian. *On Being Involved.* Denville, New Jersey: Dimension Books, 1970.

van Kaam, Adrian. *Living Creatively.* Denville, New Jersey: Dimension Books, 1972.

van Kaam, Adrian. *On Being Yourself.* Denville, New Jersey: Dimension Books, 1972.

van Kaam, Adrian, ed. "Conflict and Change." *Humanitas* 10 (2). Pittsburgh: Duquesne University Press, 1974.

van Kaam, Adrian, ed., "Silence and Saying." *Humanitas* 11 (2). Denville, New Jersey: Dimension Books, 1975.

van Kaam, Adrian, ed. "The Value of the Human." *Humanitas* 15 (2). Pittsburgh: Duquesne University Press, 1979.

van Kaam, Adrian, ed., "The Freedom of the Human." *Humanitas* 15 (3). Pittsburgh: Duquesne University Press, 1979.

van Kaam, Adrian, ed. "Spirituality and Originality." *Studies in Formative Spirituality* 1 (1). Pittsburgh: Duquesne University Press, 1980.

van Kaam, Adrian, ed. "Spirituality and the Desert Experience." *Studies in Formative Spirituality* 1 (2). Pittsburgh: Duquesne University Press, 1980.

van Kaam, Adrian, Bert van Croonenburg, and Susan Muto. *The Emergent Self.* Wilkes-Barre, Pennsylvania: Dimension Books, 1968.

van Kaam, Adrian, Bert van Croonenburg, and Susan Muto. *The Participant Self.* Vol. I and II. Denville, New Jersey: Dimension Books, 1969.

Van Perusen, Cornelius. *A Phenomenology and Reality.* Pittsburgh: Duquesne University Press, 1972.

von Bertalanffy, Ludwig. *General System Theory: Foundations, Development, Applications.* New York: George Braziller, 1968.

Watts, Alan W. *The Wisdom of Insecurity.* New York: Pantheon Books, 1951.

Watzlawick, Paul. *An Anthology of Human Communication, Text and Tape.* Palo Alto, California: Science and Behavior Books, 1974.

Watzlawick, Paul. *How Real is Real?* New York: Vintage Books, 1977.

Watzlawick, Paul. *The Language of Change.* New York: Basic Books, 1978.

Watzlawick, Paul, Janet Beavin, and Don D. Jackson. *Pragmatics of Human Communication: A Study of Interactional Patterns, Pathologies, and Paradoxes.* New York: W. W. Norton, 1967.

Watzlawick, Paul, John Weakland, and Richard Fisch. *Change: Principles of Problem Formation and Problem Resolution.* New York: W. W. Norton, 1974.

Werkmeister, W. H. *Historical Spectrum of Value Theories.* Lincoln, Nebraska: Johnson Publishing Co., 1970.

Wertenbaker, Lael Tucker. *Death of a Man.* Boston: Beacon Press, 1974.

White, John, and Stanley Krippner, eds. *Future Science.* New York: Doubleday, 1977.

Whitehead, Alfred North. *Modes of Thought.* New York: The Free Press, 1938.

Whitehead, Alfred North. *Science and the Modern World.* New York: Macmillan, 1925.

Whitehead, Alfred North. *Process and Reality.* New York: The Free Press, 1969.

Wolf, Richard. *Evaluation in Education.* New York: Praeger Publishers, Praeger Special Studies, 1979.

Zaner, Richard, and Don Ihde. *Phenomenology and Existentialism.* New York: G. P. Putnam's Sons, 1973.

Index

Administering Nursing
Service Practicum
(course), 139-142
Administrative Process
(course), 137-139
Administrator-nurse process,
111

Baker family, 55
Bandler, Richard, 47, 49
Becoming, 25, 29, 30, 31,
39, 62, 99
alternative ways, 13
Being and non-being, 19, 27,
57
Bronowski, Jacob, 174
Bruteau, Beatrice, 43, 61
Buber, Martin, 54

Certainty-uncertainty, 61
Change, 31, 41, 58, 62
first- and second order,
63-65
Choice, 21, 27, 29, 30, 39,
42, 45, 49, 56
Class visitation form, 169
Coconstitution, 7, 14, 19,
20, 22, 25, 26, 28,
30, 48, 55, 70, 73, 88
Coexistence, 7, 19, 20, 22,
25, 26, 33, 70
Comparative Studies in
Nursing Leadership
(course), 146-148
Complementarity, 7, 13,
15, 22, 70

Concept Development and
Theory Evolution
(course), 114-116
Conceptual approach, 4
Conceptual systems, 4
Conflict, 58
Conformity-nonconformity,
60
Connecting-separating, 31,
41, 53-55, 67, 69, 71,
73, 80, 81, 90
Contextual situations, 87-89
Copernicus, 5, 6
Cotranscending with the
possibles, 41, 55-68
Course end data, 155-159
Courses:
conceptual focus, 112-151
descriptions, 112-151
electives, 108, 142-153
evaluations, 151-172
focal, 106, 112-122
role, 107, 133-151
sequence, 108-110
subsidiary, 106, 122-133
see also Course titles
Course titles:
Administering Nursing
Service Practicum,
139-142
Administrative Process, 137-
139
Comparative Studies in
Nursing Leadership,
146-148
Concept Development and

Theory Evolution, 114-116

Curriculum Process, 133-135

Family, 120-122

Family-Nurse Process I, 122-124

Family-Nurse Process II, 124-126

Family-Nurse Process III, 126-128

Family Life Experiences, 130-132

Family Patterns of Relating, 128-130

Leadership Foundations, 116-118

Nursing Leadership and Health Care Systems, 148-149

Nursing Leadership and Institutions of Higher Learning, 149-151

Nursing Leadership and Technological Resources, 142-143

Nursing Research I, 118-120

Nursing Research II, 132-133

Nursing Science: Man-Living-Health, 112-114

Political Issues in Nursing Leadership, 114-145

Teaching Nursing Practicum, 135-137

Curriculum plan:
based on Man-Living-Health, 96-112
course plan, sample, 105-108
elements of, 91-96
evaluation process, 94-96

financial evaluation, 95
focal courses, 106
goals, 91-92, 93, 100-105
instructional strategies, 110-112
philosophy, 91-92, 93

Curriculum Process (course), 133-135

Daly family, 61-62

Darwin, Charles, 5

Data, 94-96
financial, 171-172
process, 168
supplemental, 168-171

Dilthey, Wilhelm, 11, 42, 44, 57, 63

Doctoral curriculum, 77

Dubos, Rene, 40

Education:
implications for, 90-172
theory, research, and practice, 77

Elective courses, 108, 142-153

Ellis, Rosemary, 3

Enabling-limiting, 50, 53, 69, 71, 73, 79, 81

Energy, 27, 28, 31, 33
field, 14, 15, 16, 18, 22, 25, 28, 33, 70
interchange with environment, 31, 32, 39, 57

Epilogue, 173-175

Evaluation model, sample graduate nursing program, 152-153

Evaluation plan, sample, 150-172

Evans family, 65-67

Existential-phenomenology, 4, 5, 7, 13, 18-22, 68

Facticity, 19, 21, 31

Faculty-student process, 110

Familiar-unfamiliar, 63
Family (course), 120-122
Family-nurse process, 110-111
Family-Nurse Process I (course), 122-124
Family-Nurse Process II (course), 124-126
Family-Nurse Process III (course), 126-128
Family Life Experiences (course), 130-132
Family Patterns of Relating (course), 128-130
Family situation, 83-87
Ferguson, Marilyn, 40, 63, 64, 65
Financial data, 171-172
Focal courses, 106
Four-dimensionality, 14, 17, 22, 25, 28, 30, 33, 70
Frankl, Viktor E., 40, 56

Glossary, 177-179
Goldstein, Kurt, 39
Greene, Maxine, 44
Grinder, John, 47, 49

Hall, Brian P., 45
Hall, Edward T., 47
Health, 7, 13, 14, 40, 70, 81
  focus on, 12
  as intersubjective process, 25, 32
  living, 30
  as negentropic unfolding, 33, 39
  paradigm of, 40
  as patterns of relating, 25, 26
  as relative present, 31
  as synthesis of values, 31-32, 39
Heidegger, Martin, 5, 18, 19, 20

Helicy, 7, 13, 15, 22, 70
Henderson, Virginia, 7
Historicity, 19
Homo naturus, 12
Human science, 3, 6, 11, 13, 78
Human science nursing, 7, 11, 40-41
Human subjectivity, 7, 19, 22, 70

Imaged values, 48-50, 67
Imaging, 42-44, 69, 71, 73, 78
  reflective-prereflective, 43
Input, 94
Instructional strategies, 110-112
Intentionality, 18-19, 22, 70
Introduction to the Theoretical Basis of Nursing, An, 4

Kempler, Walter, 54
King, Imogene, 4
Knowing, explicit and tacit, 43-44, 81
Kuhn, Thomas S., 6

Laing, R. D., 64
Langer, Susanne, 47, 49
Languaging, 46-50, 57, 67, 69, 71, 73, 80, 81
  values, 32
Leadership Foundations (course), 116-118
Leininger, Madeleine, 7
Leonard, George B., 51
Level indicators, 160-167
Lived experiences, 78-80
Living health, 30

Macquarrie, John, 11
Man:
  enabled and limited, 27

and environment, 16, 17,
    25, 26, 55, 56, 99
  energy interchange, 29,
    99
  and health, 7, 17
    assumptions, 25-36
  as living unity, 4, 16
  natural science view of, 12
  particulate view of, 12
  as questioning being, 43
  as sum of parts, 7
Man-Living-Health, theory of,
    4, 5, 8, 13, 14, 18, 21,
    25, 33, 39, 68, 72
  assumptions, 25-36, 70,
    98-99
    concept-assumption
      interface, 35
    evolution of, 34
    with related concepts, 36
  cadence, 50
  curriculum plan based on,
    96-112
  empirical aspects, 77-172
  evolution of, 70
  paradigm of, 11-13
  practice implications, 80-
    90
  principles, concepts, and
    structures, 13-21, 39-73
  research implications, 77-
    80
  theoretical structure, 68-
    69, 72
Man-world dialectic, 20
Marcel, Gabriel, 56
Medical model of nursing, 12
Medical science, 12
Merleau-Ponty, Maurice, 20,
    48, 56
Metaperspective, 64
Multidimensionality, 28-29,
    41-50
Muto, Susan, 54

Natural science, 3

Natural science nursing, 3, 11
Negentropic unfolding, 25,
    33, 39, 60, 73
Newman, Margaret, 5
Nietzsche, Friedrich, 60
Nightingale, Florence, 12
Nursing:
  administrating, 108
  as human science, 7, 11,
    40-41
  medical model of, 12
  as natural science, 3, 11
  teaching, 107-108
Nursing leadership, 108
Nursing Leadership and
    Health Care Systems
    (course), 148-149
Nursing Leadership and
    Institutions of Higher
    Learning (course), 149-
    151
Nursing Leadership and Tech-
    nological Resources
    (course), 142-143
Nursing practice, 80-82, 89-
    90
Nursing program:
  conceptual framework, 93,
    100, 101
  course culture content, 93
  course descriptions, 112-
    151
  course plan, 105-108
  course sequence, 108-110
  evaluation process, 94-96
    financial, 95
  focal courses, 106
  indicators, 92
  industrial strategies, 110-
    112
  level indicators, 103-105
  objectives and goals, 92-
    93, 100-105
  philosophy, 91-92, 93, 98-
    100
  purpose, 97-98

see also Course titles
Nursing Research, 3
Nursing Research I (course), 118-120
Nursing Research II (course), 132-133
Nursing school, philosophy of, 91-92
Nursing Science: Man-Living-Health (course), 112-114

Openness, 14, 15, 16, 22, 27, 28, 32, 33, 70
Originating, 55, 59-62, 69, 73, 79, 90
Output, 94

Paradigm:
  emergence of, 6
  of man's health, 40
  nursing:
    comparison of, 14
    as human science, 6-7, 18
    as medical science, 13
Paradox, 60-61
Paterson, Josephine, 4
Pattern and organization, 17, 22, 25, 28, 30, 31, 70
Patterns of relating, 25, 26, 28, 32, 33, 39, 41, 50-55, 71, 73, 81, 82, 99
  timing and flowing, 51-52
Phenomenological method, 78
Phenomenological Movement, The, 78
Polanyi, Michael, 16, 43
Political Issues in Nursing Leadership (course), 144-145
Powering, 57-59, 69, 71, 73, 78, 89
Practice, prescientific, 4
Process, 95
  data, 168

Program graduates, sample questions, 170
Program indicators, 92-93
Ptolemaic theory, 6
Pushing-resisting, 57, 58, 59

Raths, Louise E., 45
Reality, 42, 45
Reflective-prereflective imaging, 43
Relating, patterns of, 25, 26, 28, 32, 33, 39, 41, 50-55, 71, 73, 81, 82, 99
  timing and flowing, 51-52
Research implications, 77-80
Resonancy, 7, 13, 15, 22, 70
Revealing-concealing, 50, 52-53, 67, 69, 71, 73, 78, 81, 89
Riehl, Joan, 4
Rogers, Marsha E., 4, 5, 6, 7, 13, 14, 16, 17, 25, 51, 68, 70
  principles, tenets, and concepts of, 7-8, 13-22, 33
Role elective courses, 142-153
Roy, Callista, 4

Sample course descriptions, 112-151
Sample evaluation plan, 150-172
Sapir, Edward, 47
Sartre, Jean-Paul, 5, 21
Schutz, Albert, 44
Situated freedom, 7, 19, 20, 22, 28, 30, 32, 70
Space-time, 29
Speaking, 47
Speigelberg, Herbert, 78
Structuring meaning multi-dimensionally, 42-50,

67, 69, 71, 73, 81
Student characteristics,
    sample form, 154-155
Student-group process, 111-
    112
Student-student process, 111
Supervisors, sample questions,
    170-171
Supplemental data, 168-171
Synergistic man, 27, 33
Synergy, 29, 32

Taylor family, 83-89
  decision making pattern
    in, 87
Teacher-student process, 111
Teaching Nursing Practicum
    (course), 135-137
Tension, 58
Themes, 93
Theoretical structure, 68, 72
  emergence of, 69

Tillich, Paul, 57
Toben, Robert, 42
Transforming, 55, 62-69, 71,
    73, 80, 90

Unitary man, 7, 16, 33, 39

Valued images, 46
Valuing, 45-46, 69, 71, 73,
    81
van Croonenburg, Bert, 55
van den Berg, J. H., 62, 78
van Kaam, Adrian, 54, 60
von Bertalanffy, Ludwig, 47

Watzlawick, Paul, 47, 48, 64,
    65
Wolf, Richard M., 94
Worldview, 43, 44, 45, 48-
    49, 58-59, 62, 65

Zderad, Loretta, 4